It's Such A Beautiful Day Outside!

Written and Illustrated
by Eman Attaya

ISBN: 9798675674725

To my family who makes everything possible.

Special thanks to my mother Adila Attaya for her insightful artistic and architectural recommendations concerning this book.

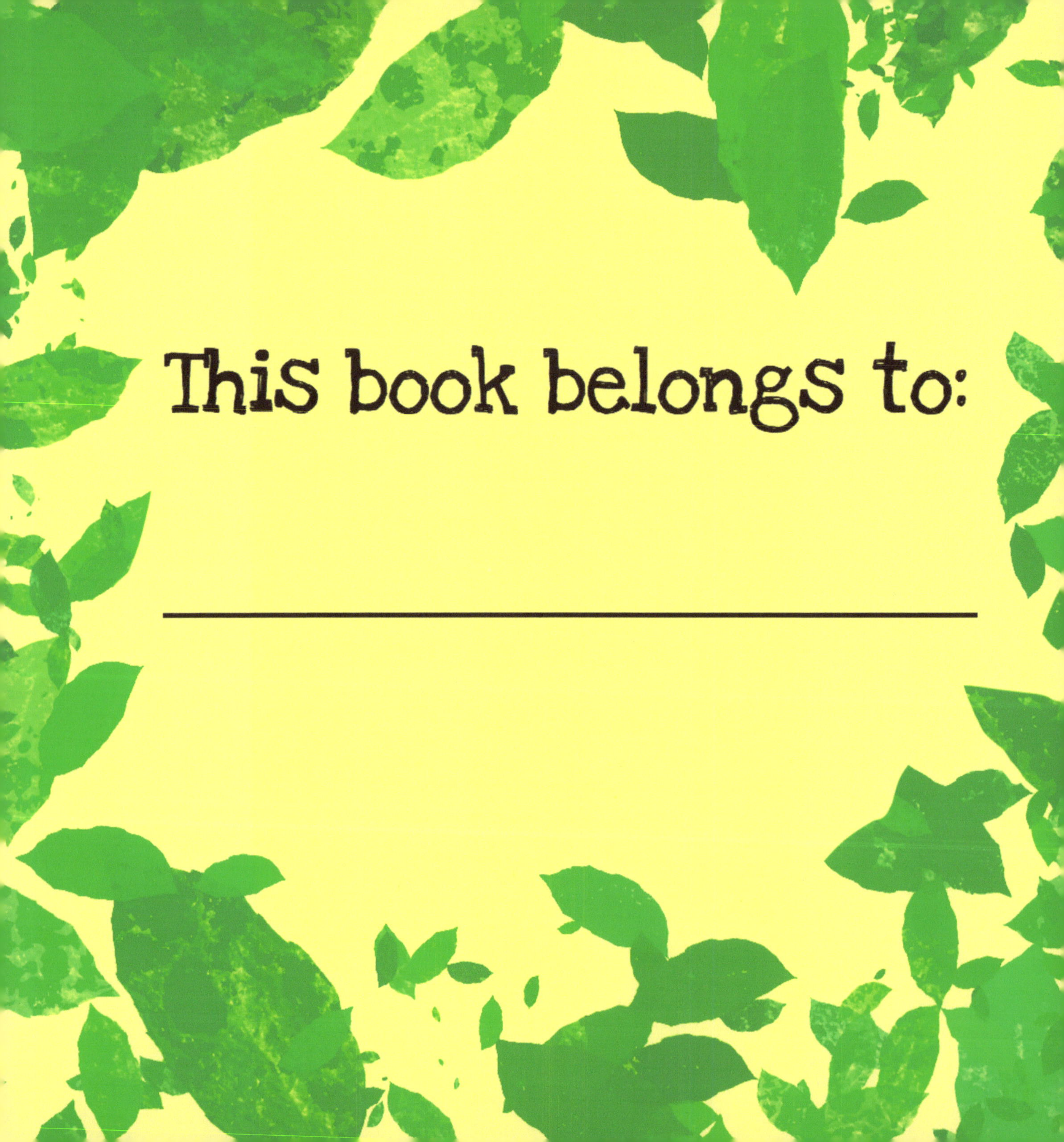

This book belongs to:

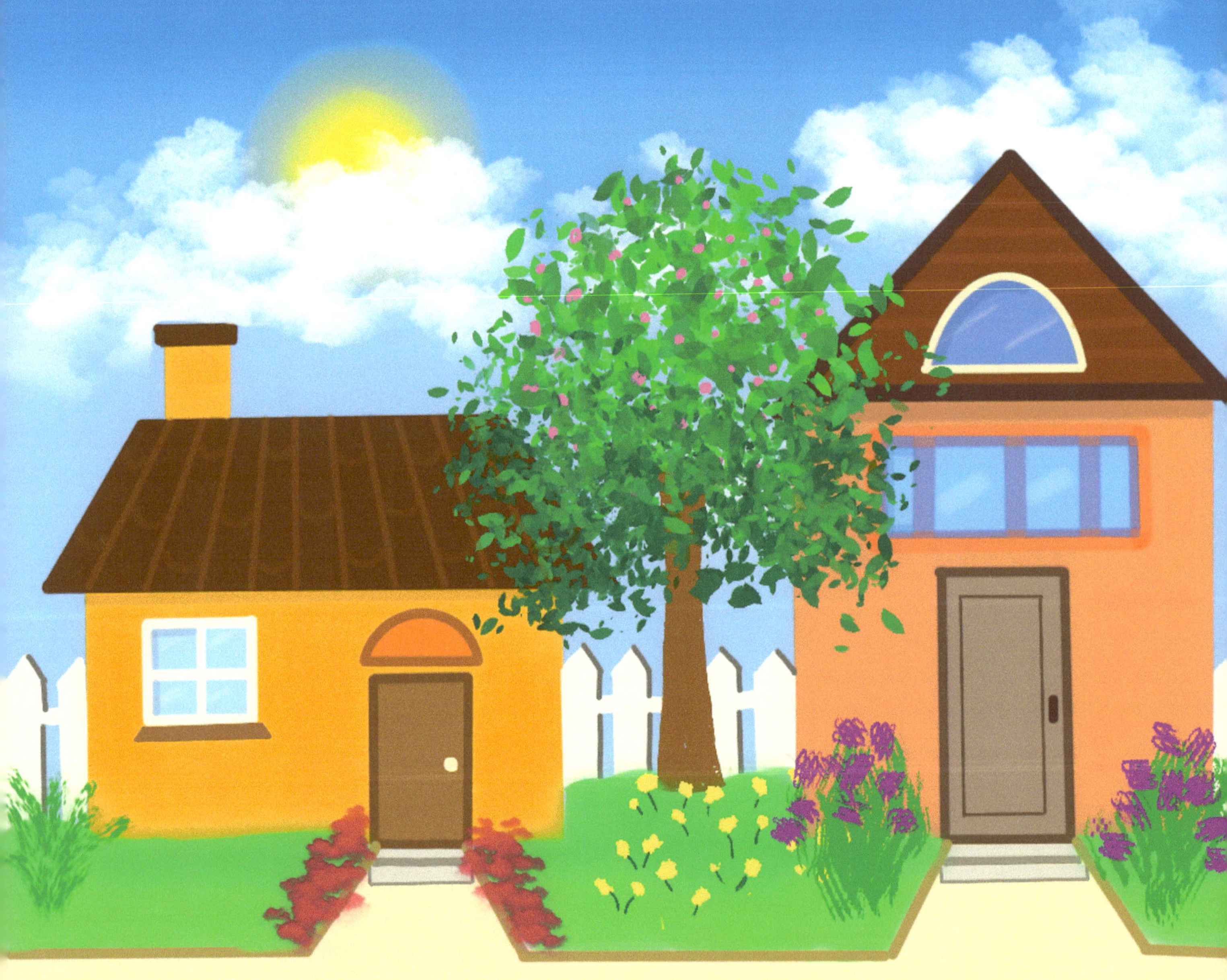
It's such a beautiful day outside!

There is no need to hide inside.

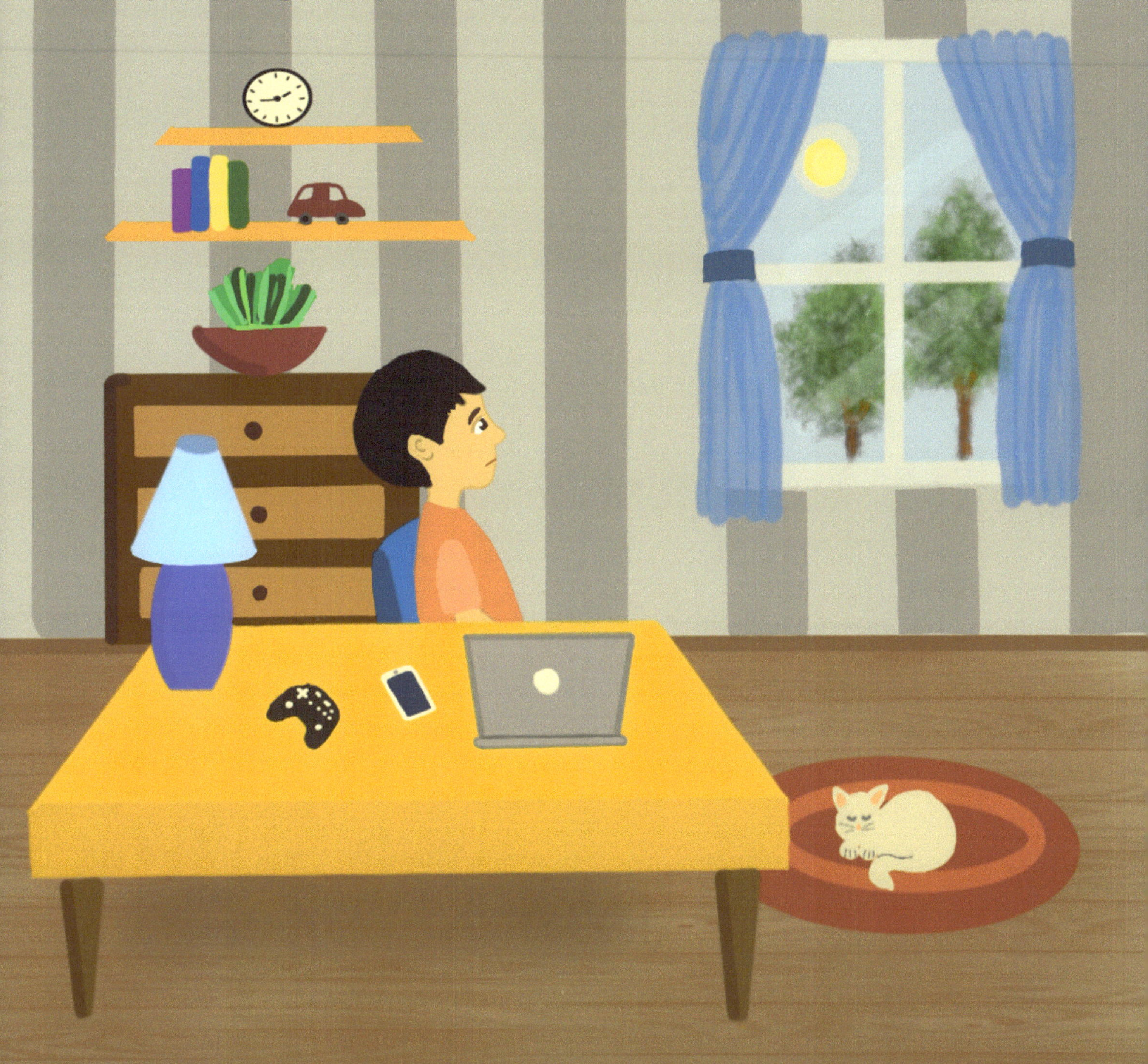

I'll put my phone and games aside

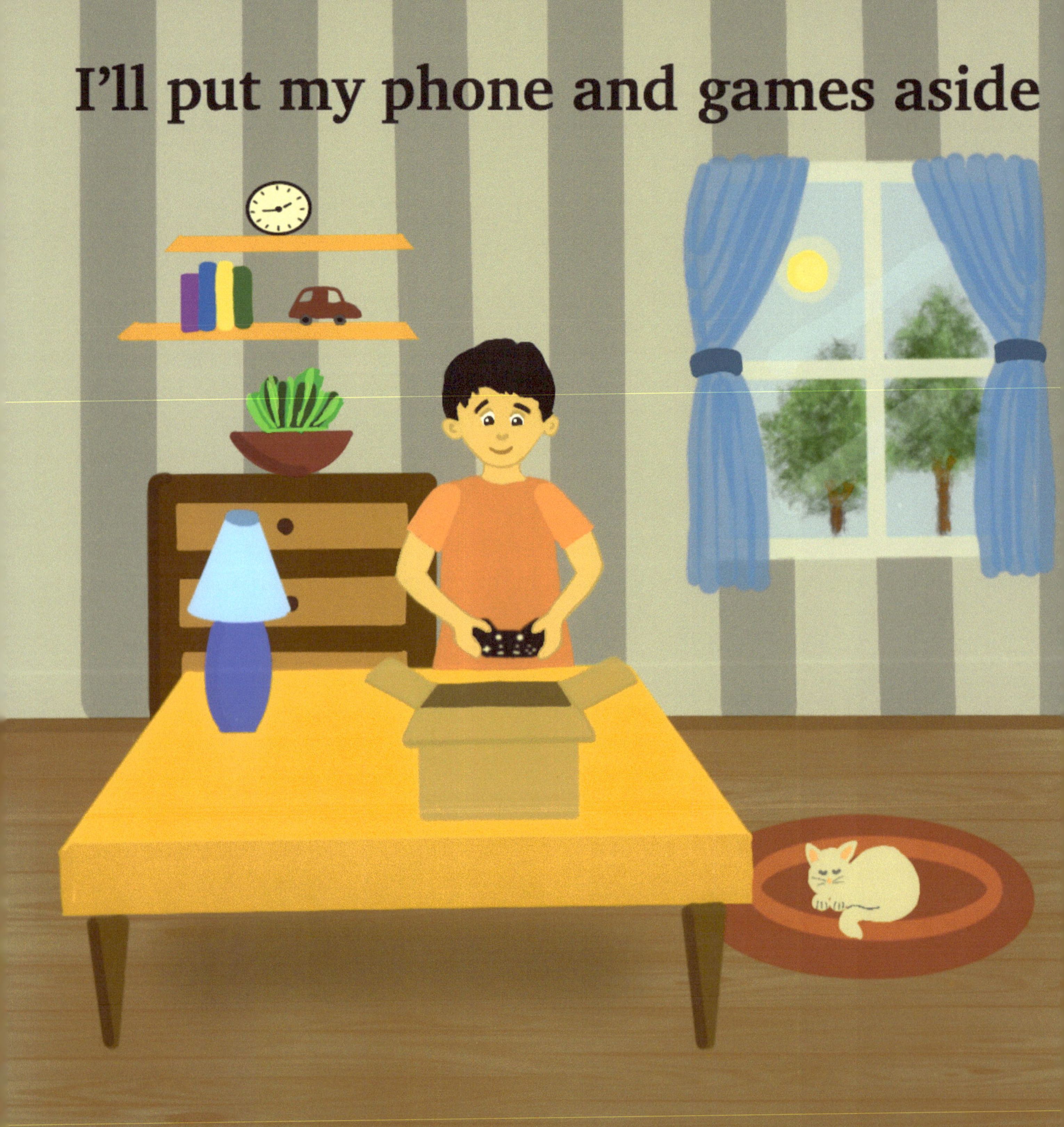

And take my bike for a lovely ride.

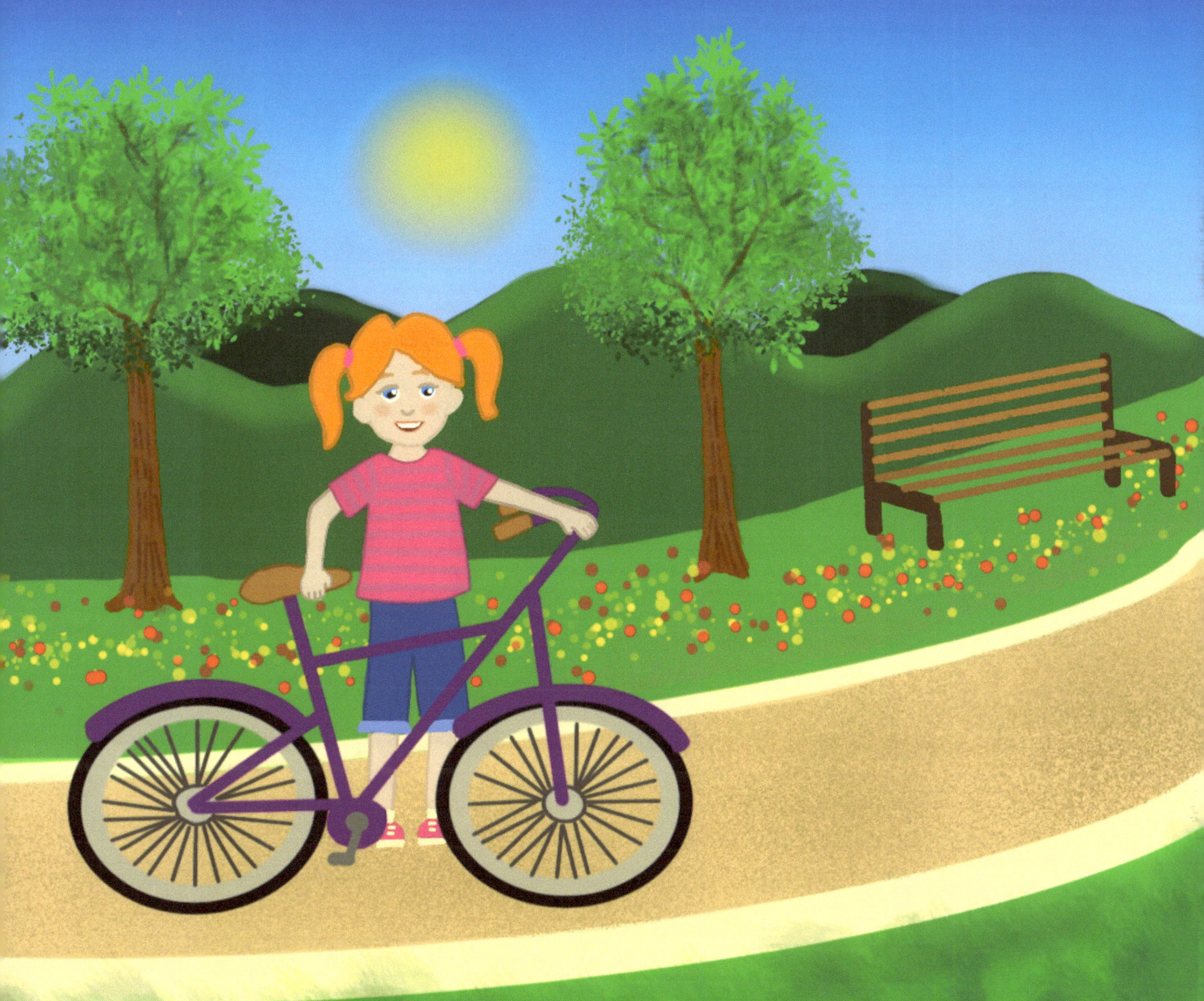

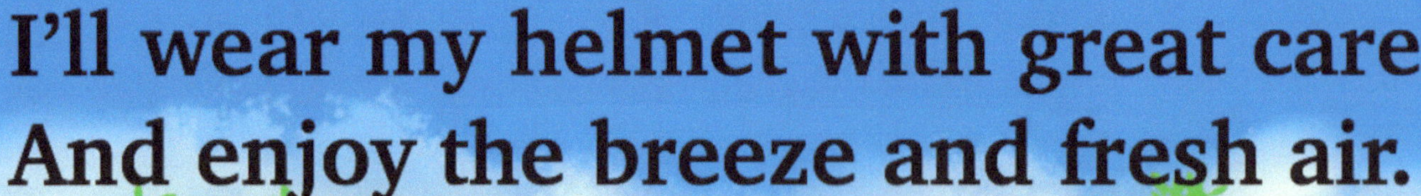

I'll wear my helmet with great care
And enjoy the breeze and fresh air.

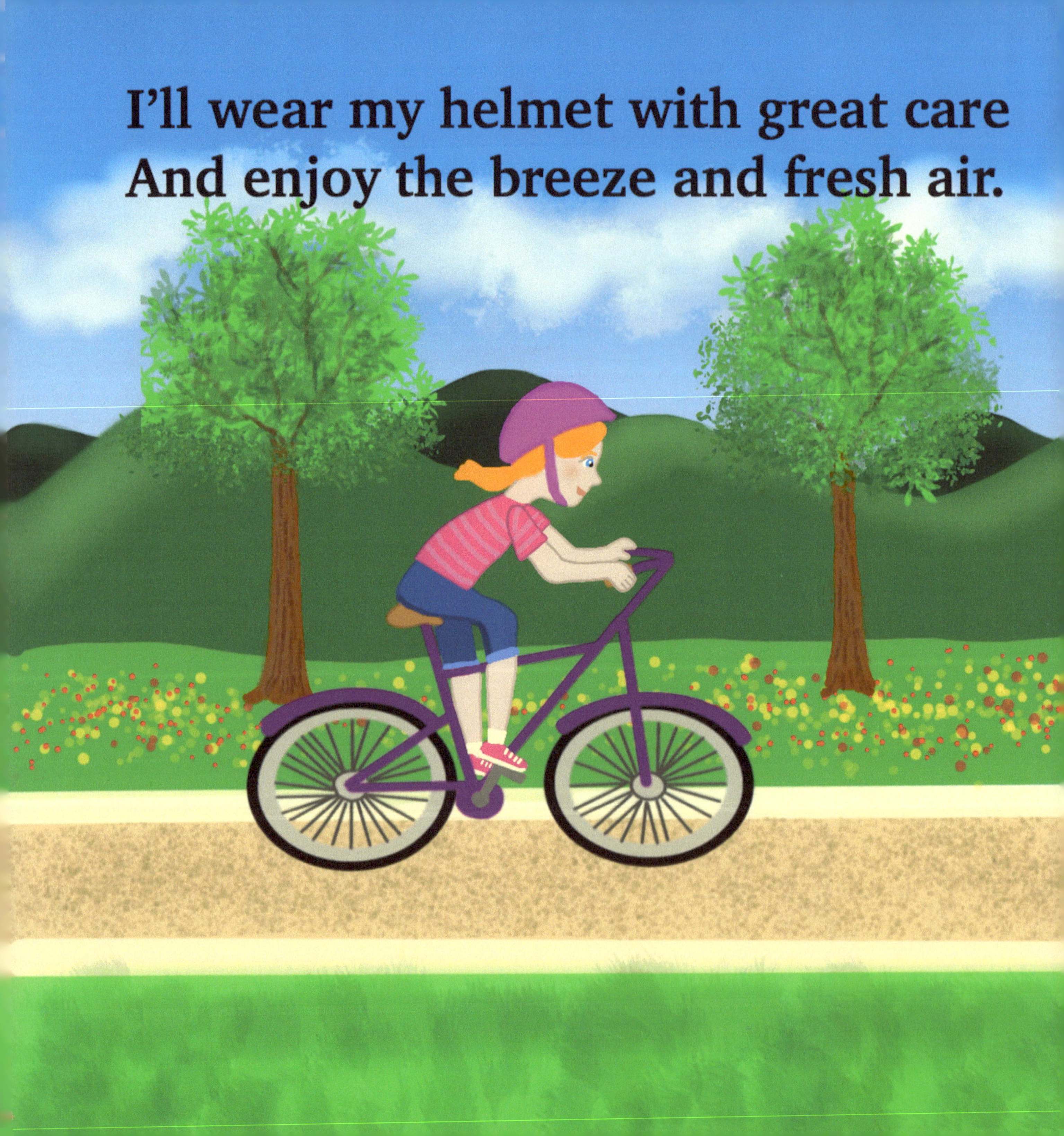

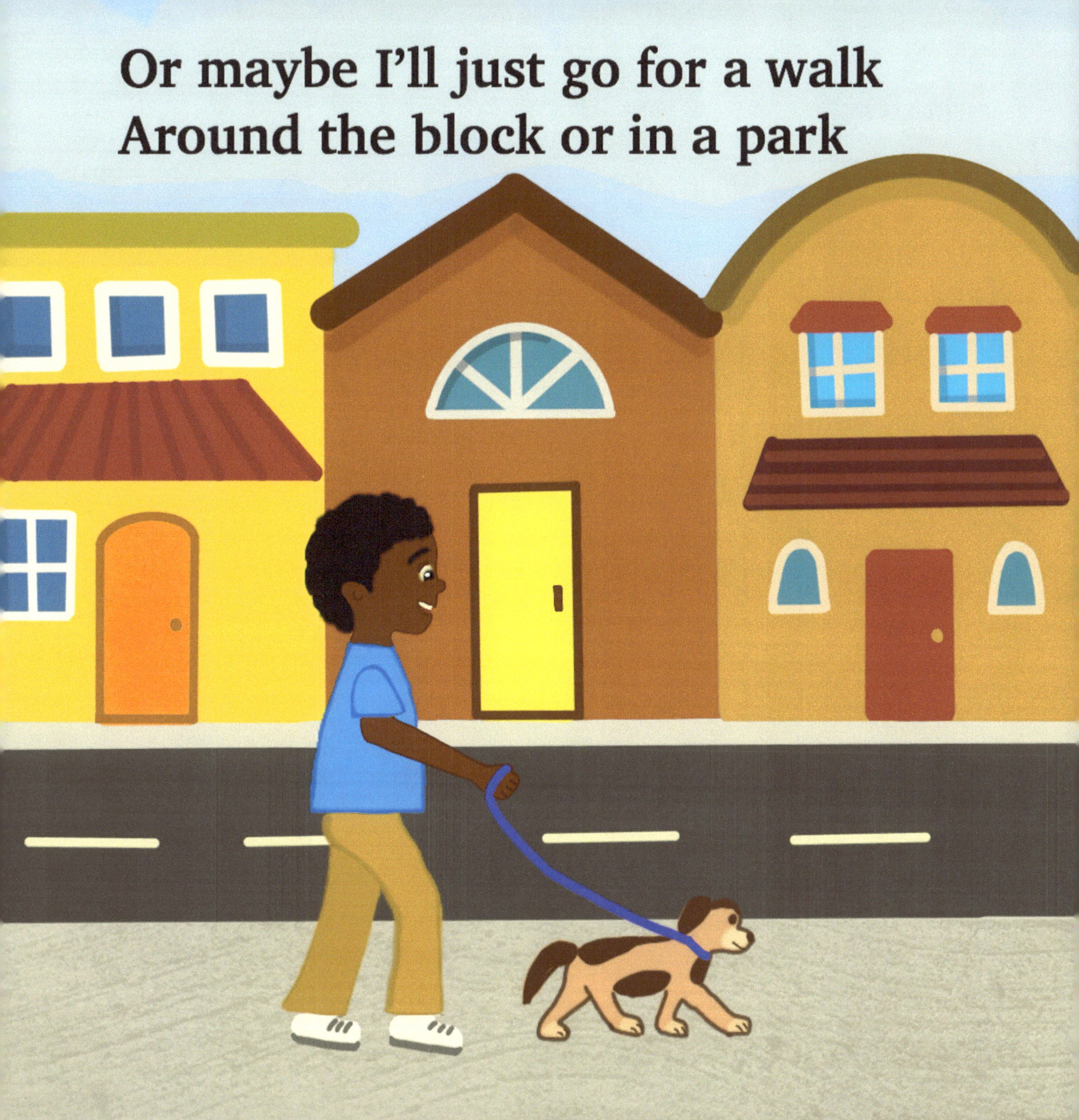
Or maybe I'll just go for a walk
Around the block or in a park

With family and friends and we can talk

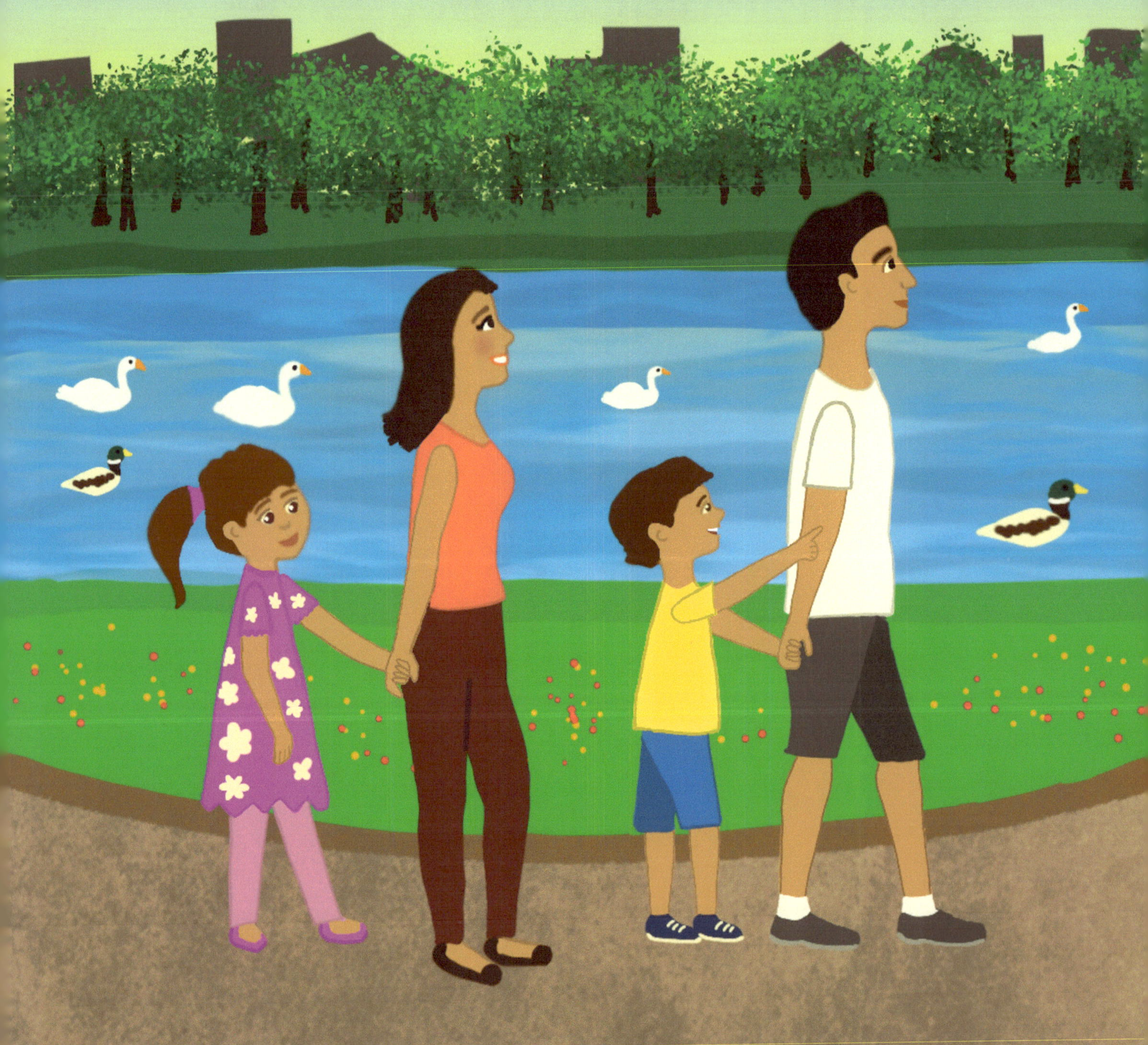

And see the dogs jump, run, and bark.

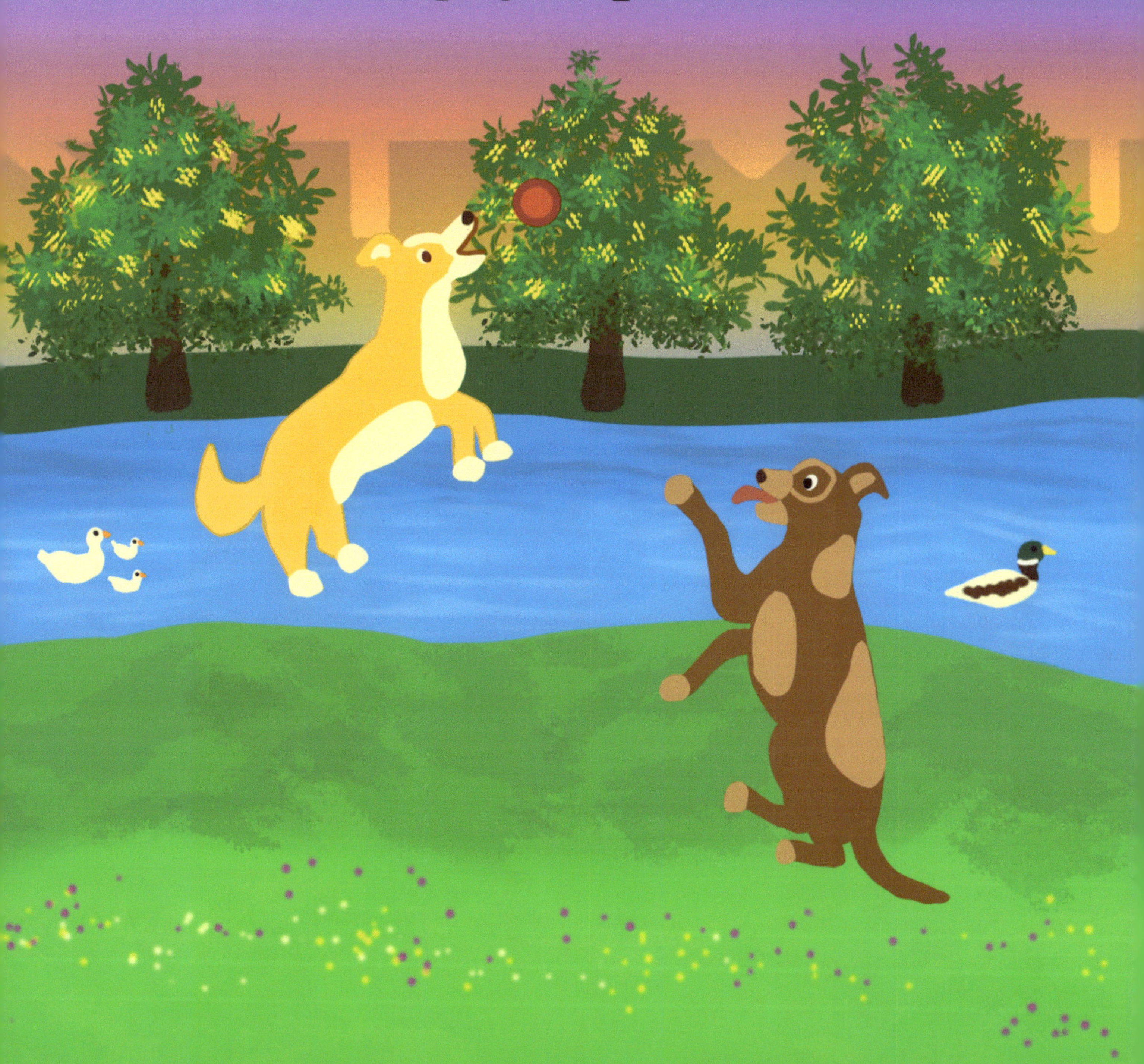

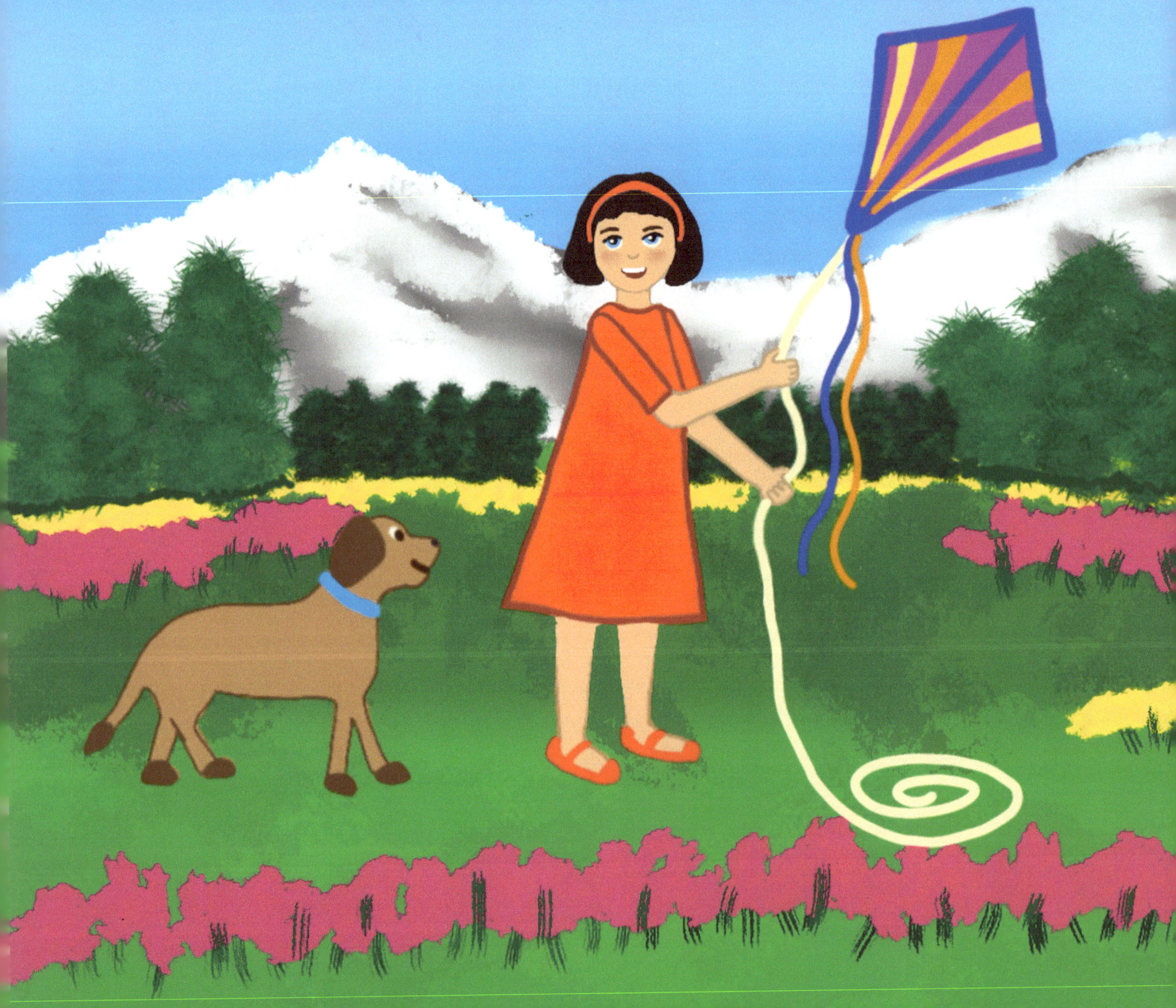

And if there's wind, I'll fly a kite,
See it soar and then take flight

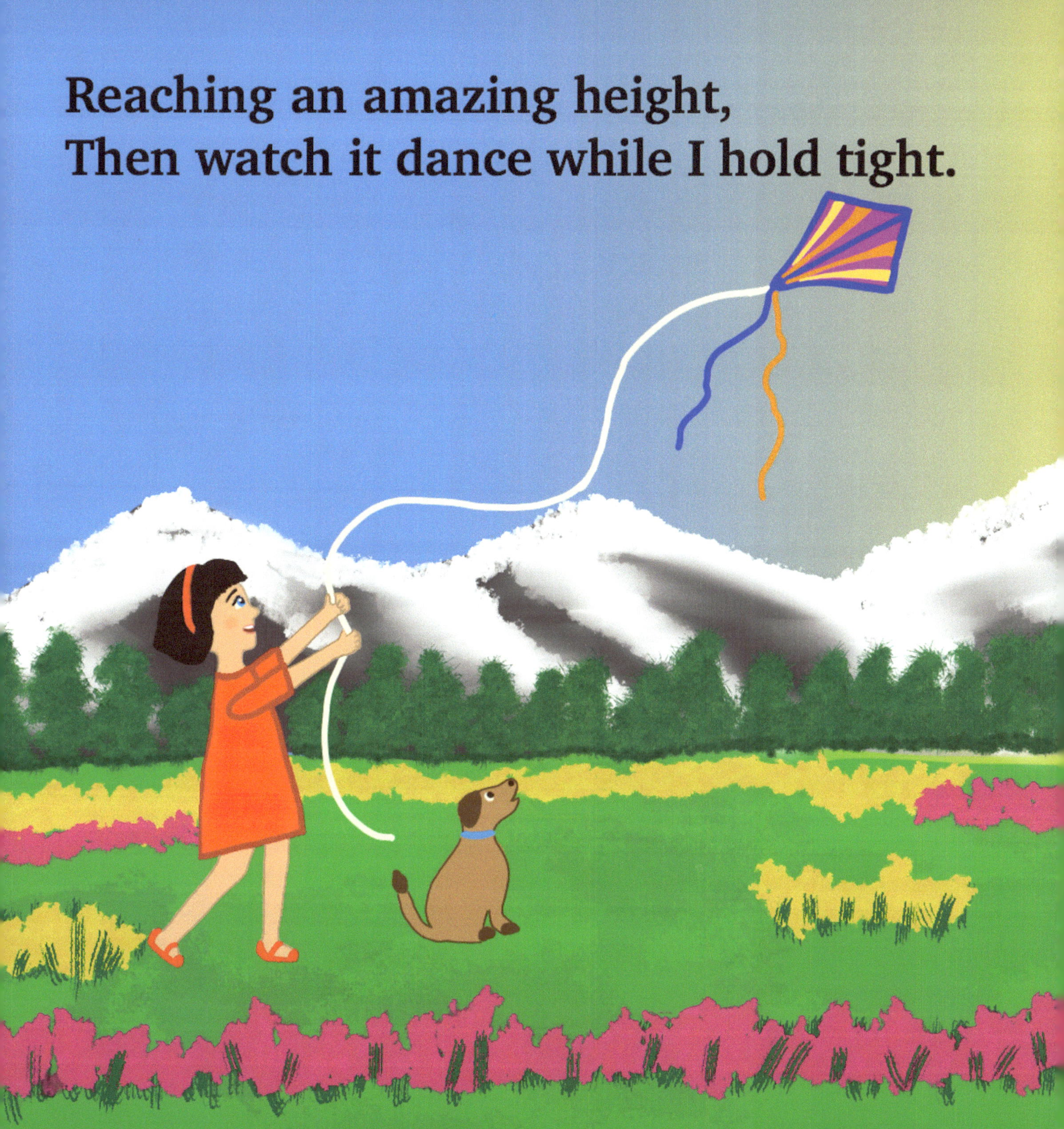
Reaching an amazing height,
Then watch it dance while I hold tight.

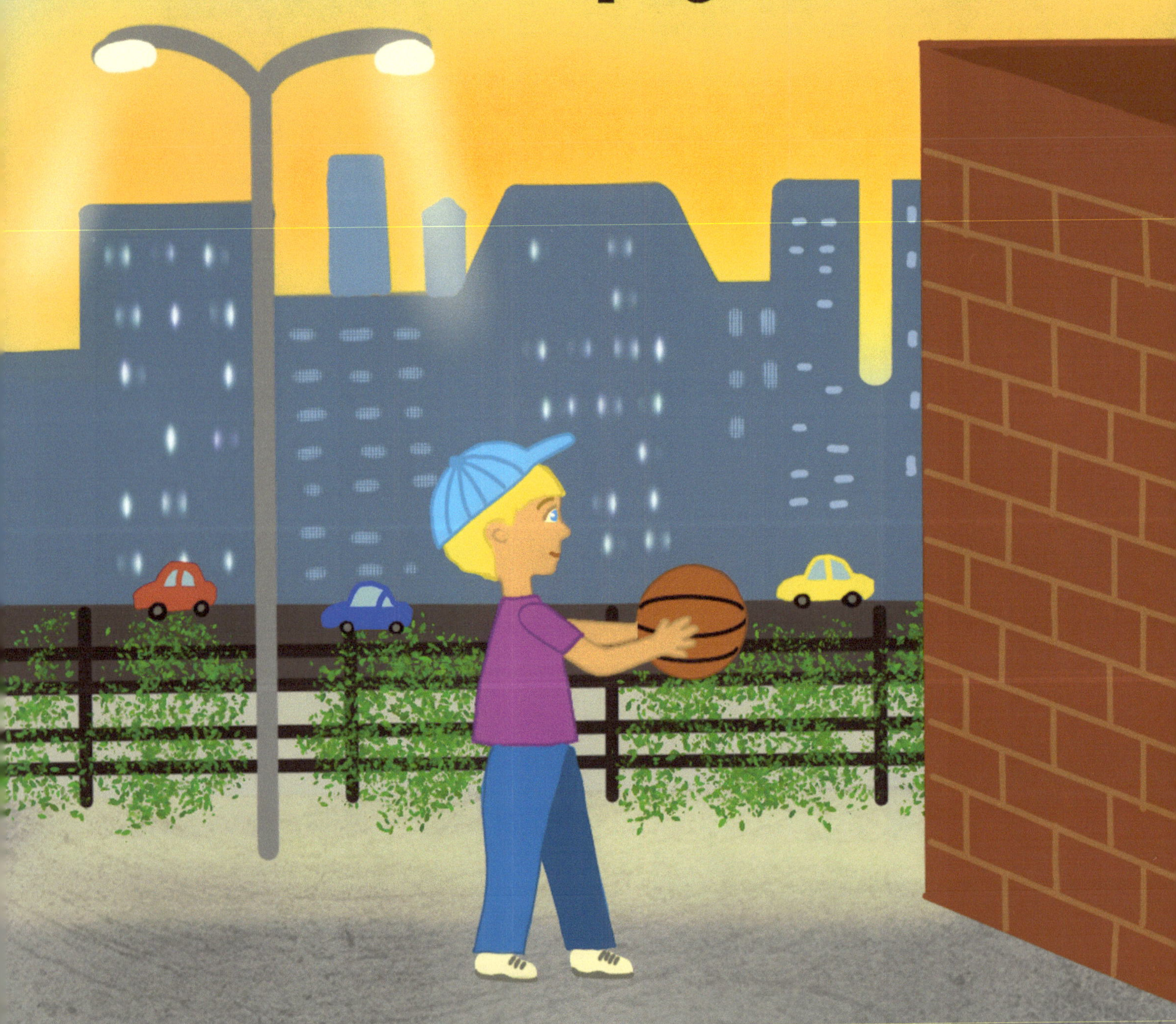
Or maybe I'll just grab a ball
And bounce it up against a wall

Play with others tossing it around

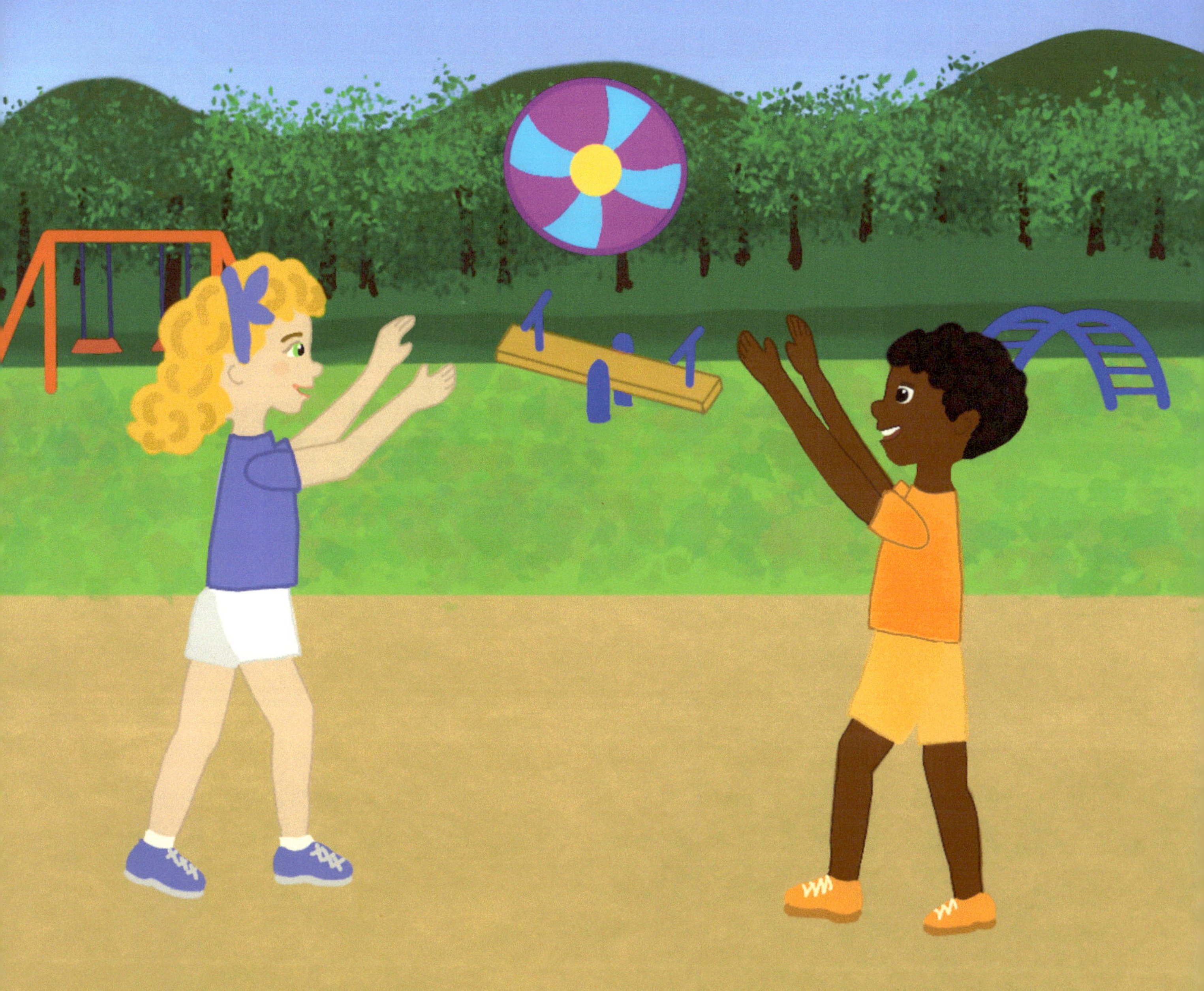

Kicking it up and off the ground.

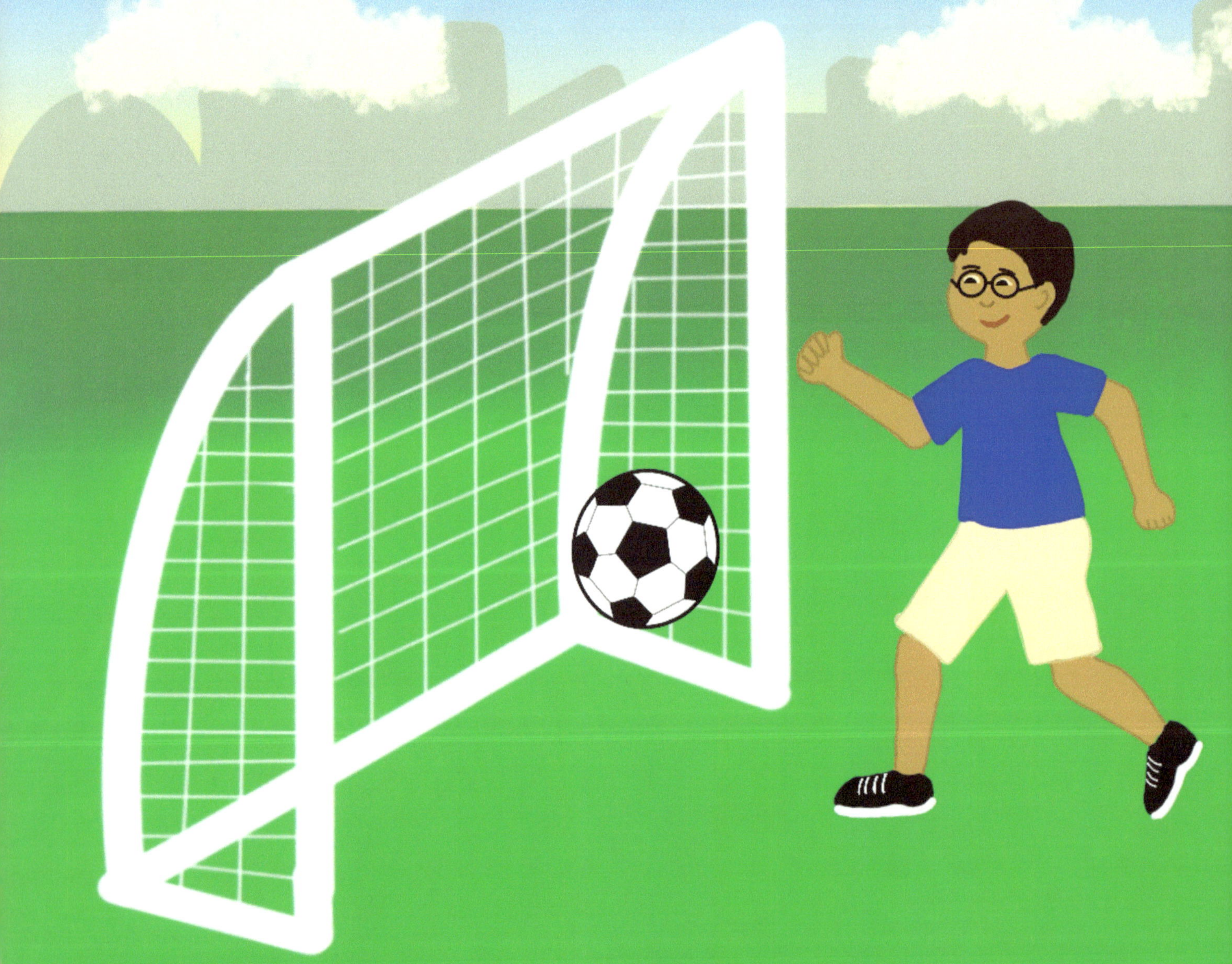

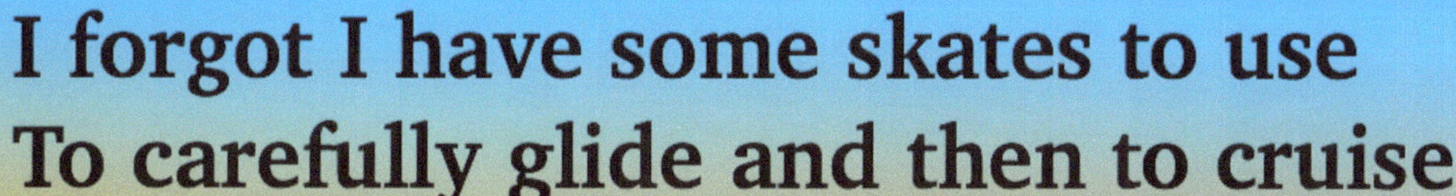

I forgot I have some skates to use
To carefully glide and then to cruise

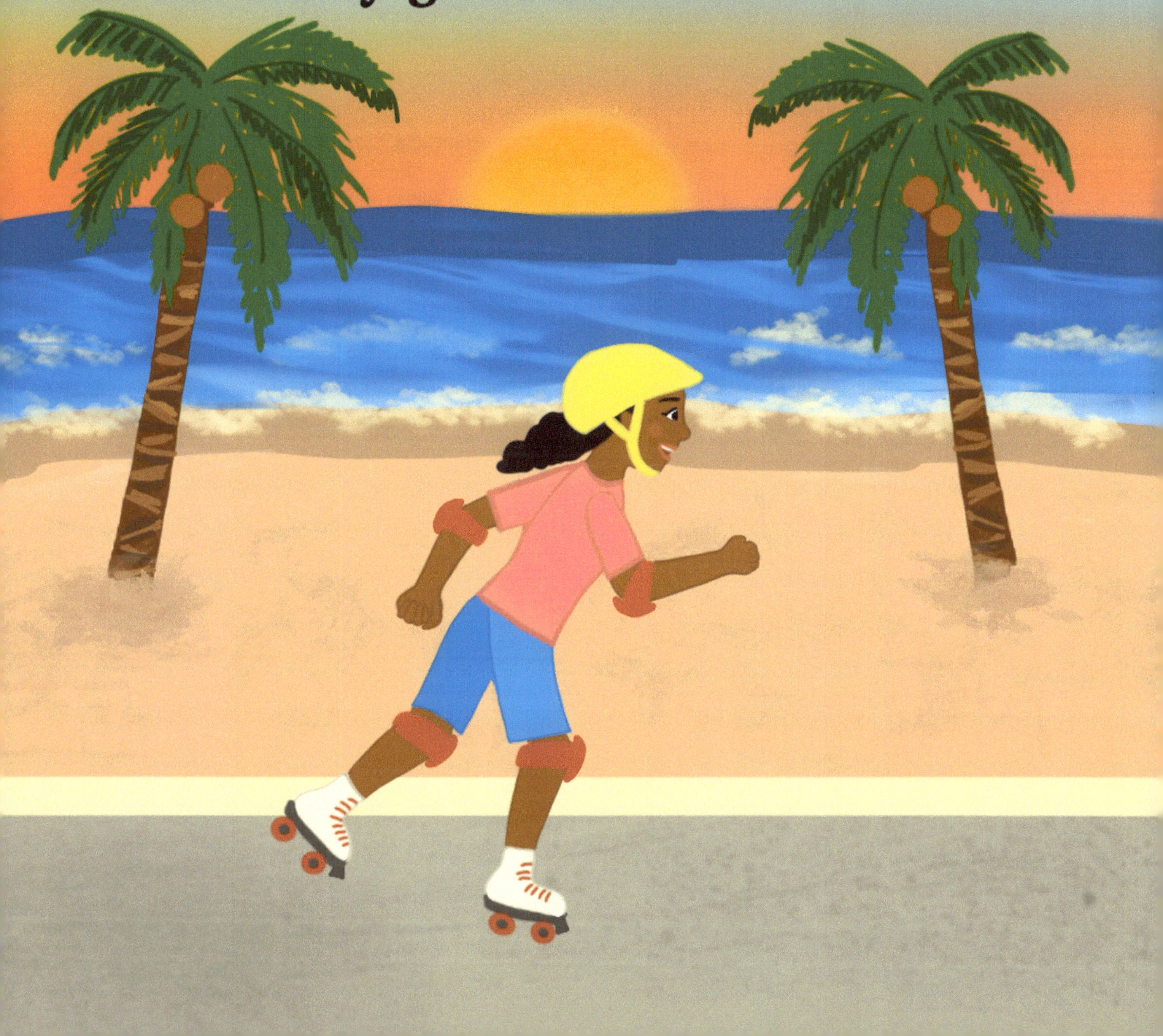

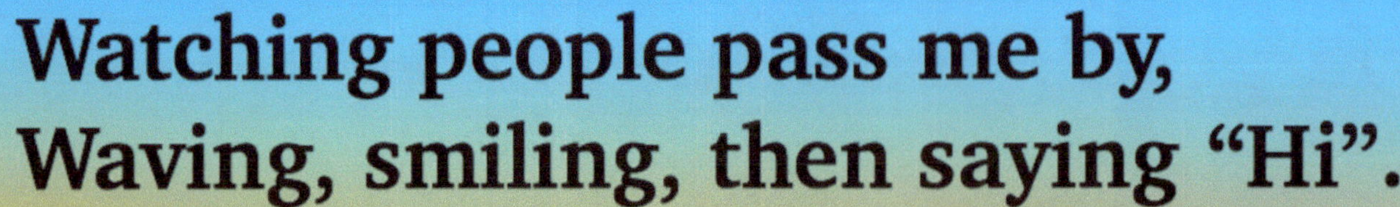

Watching people pass me by,
Waving, smiling, then saying "Hi".

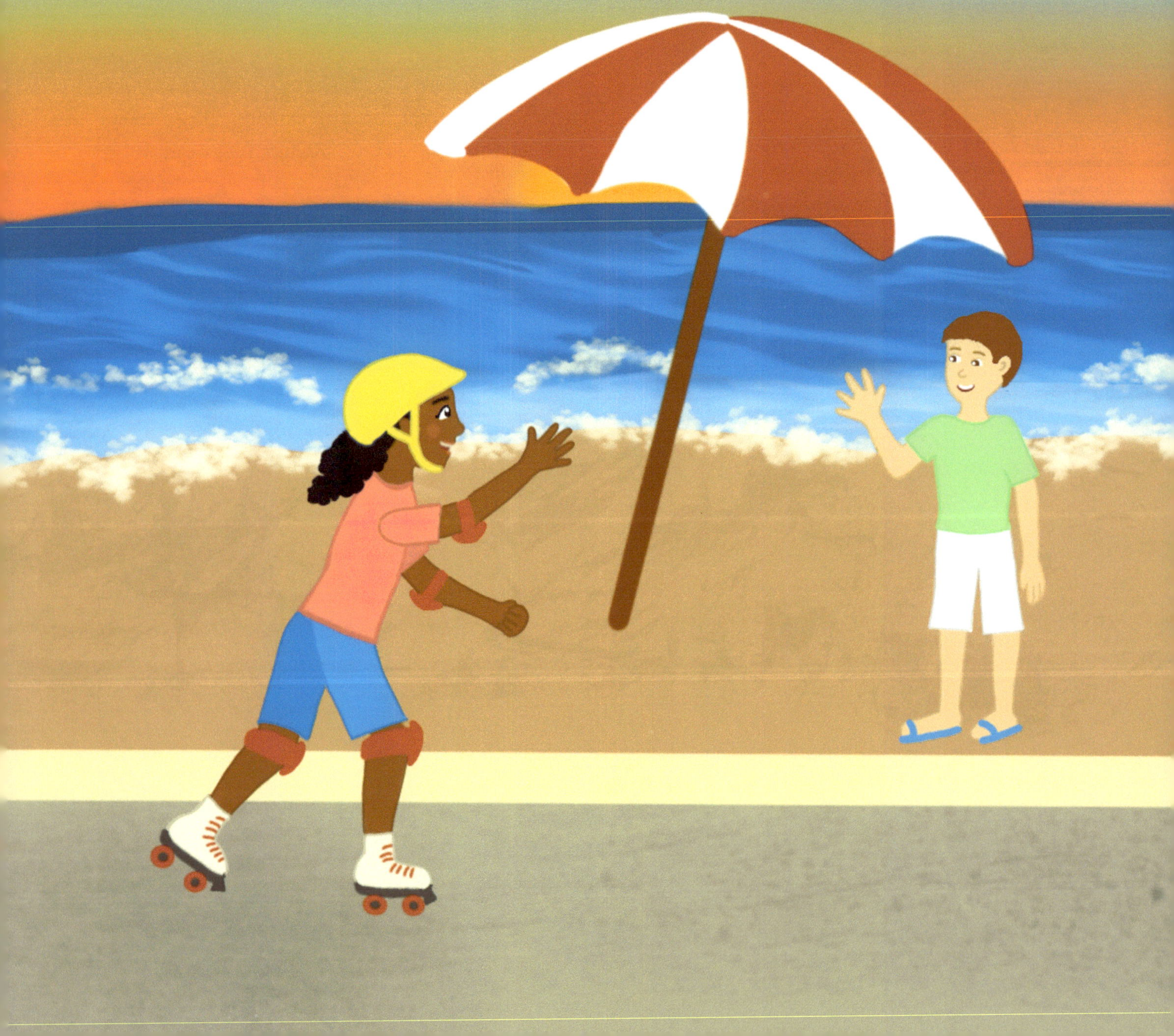

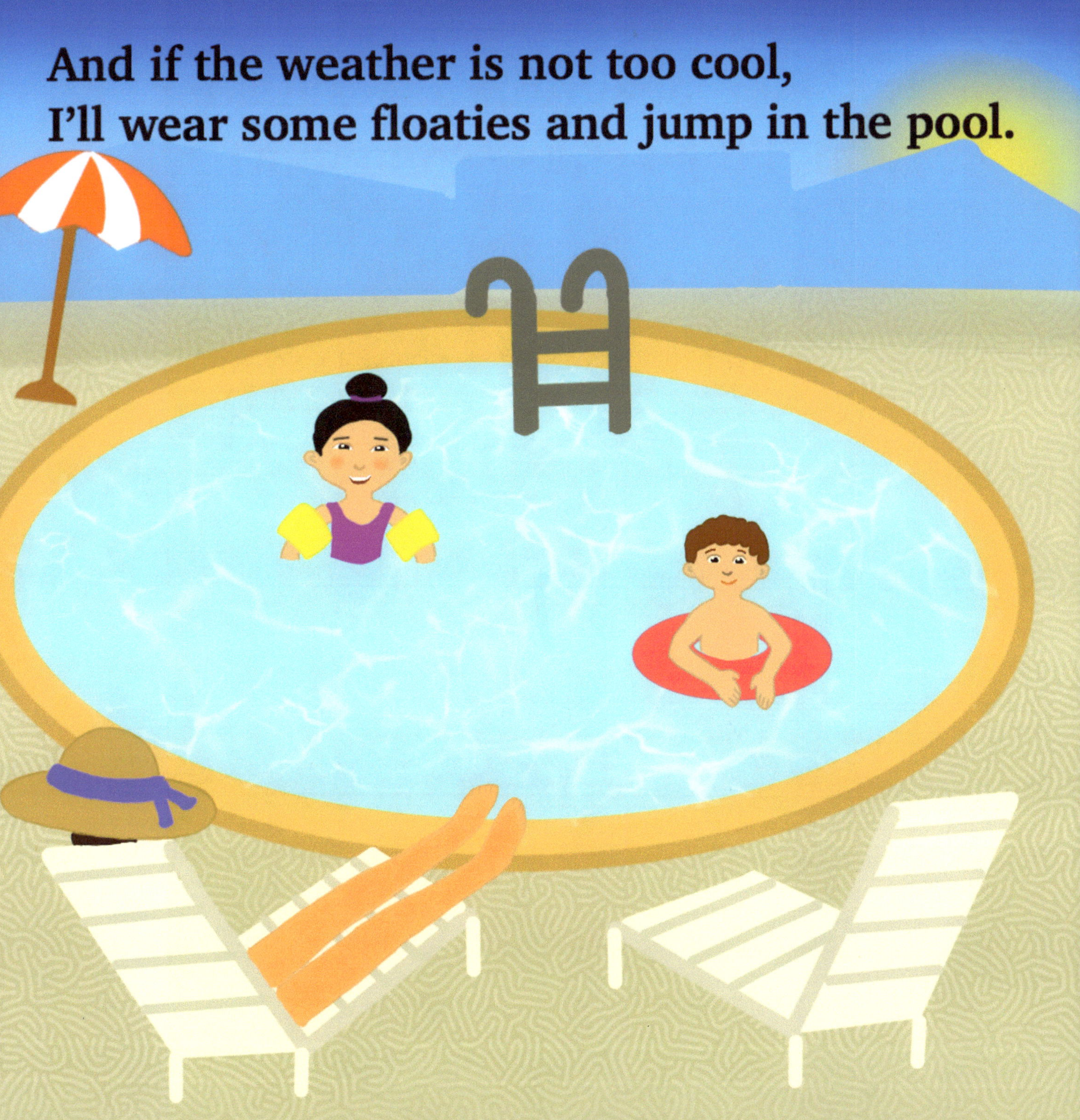
And if the weather is not too cool,
I'll wear some floaties and jump in the pool.

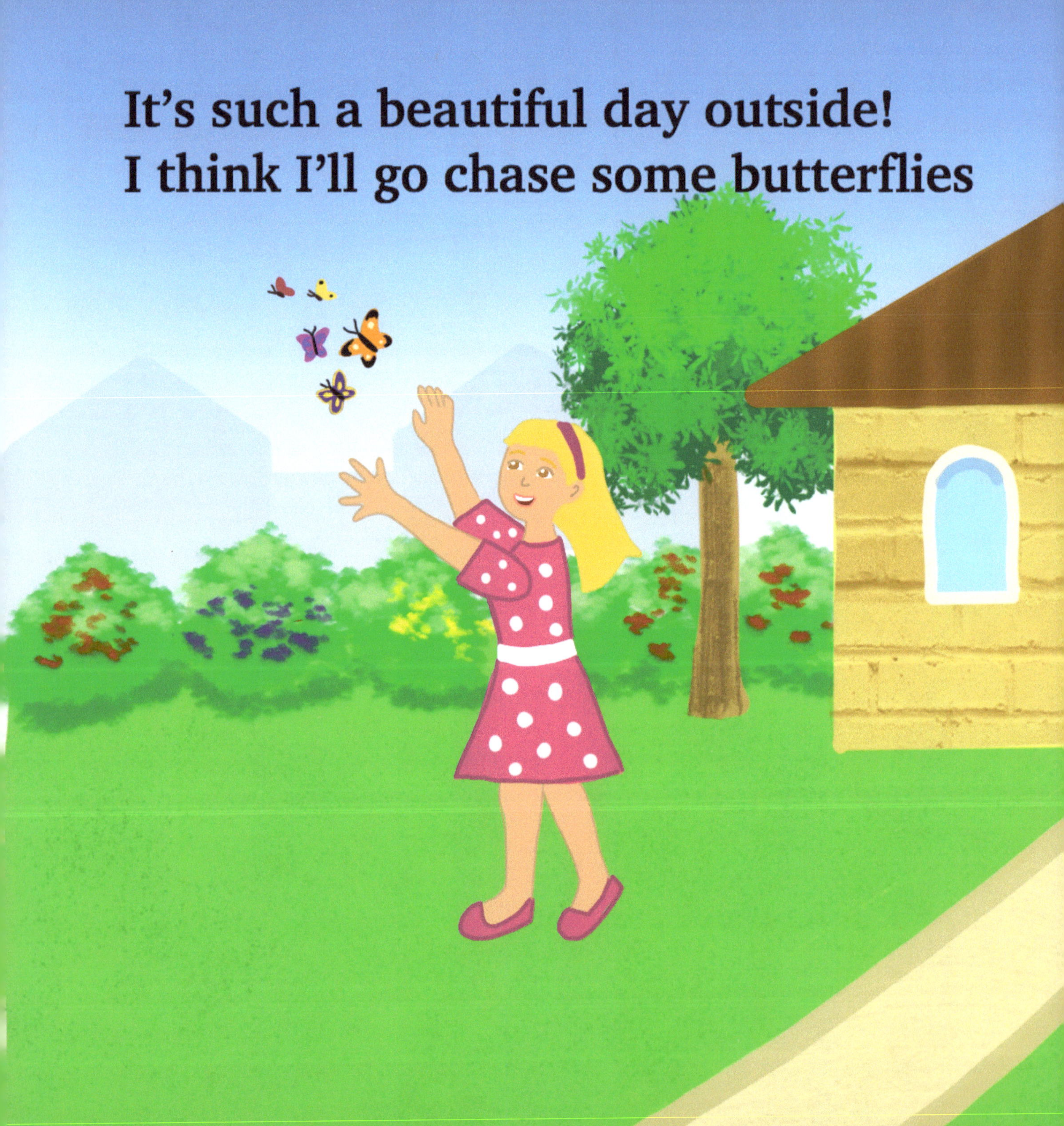
It's such a beautiful day outside!
I think I'll go chase some butterflies

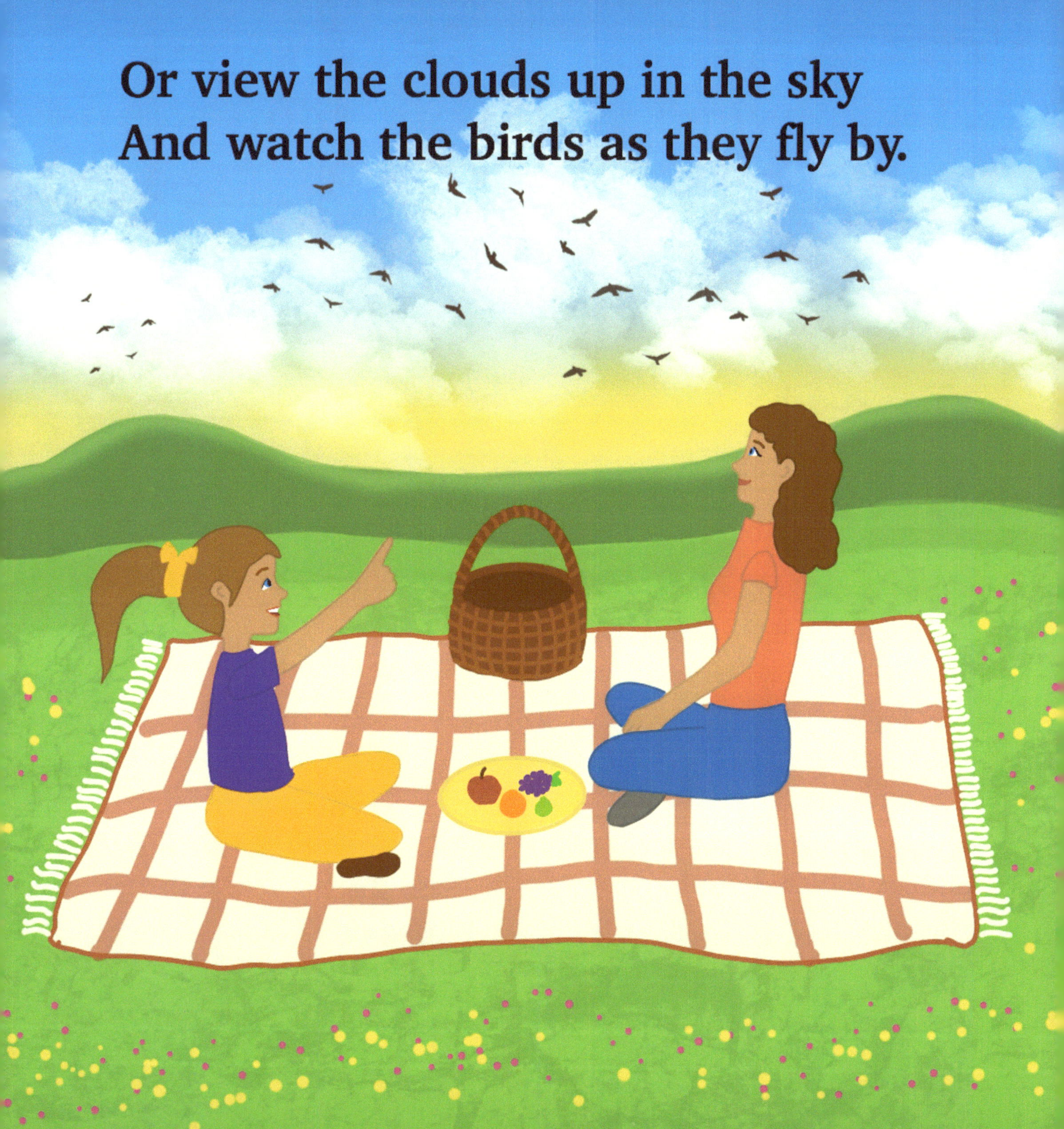
Or view the clouds up in the sky
And watch the birds as they fly by.

Or maybe I will plant some seeds

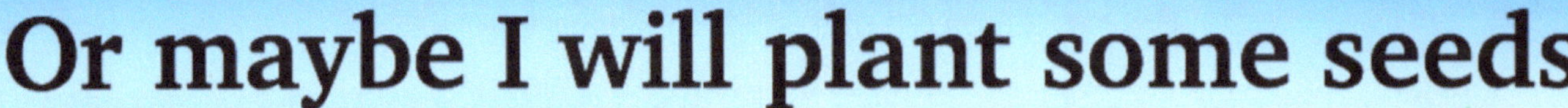

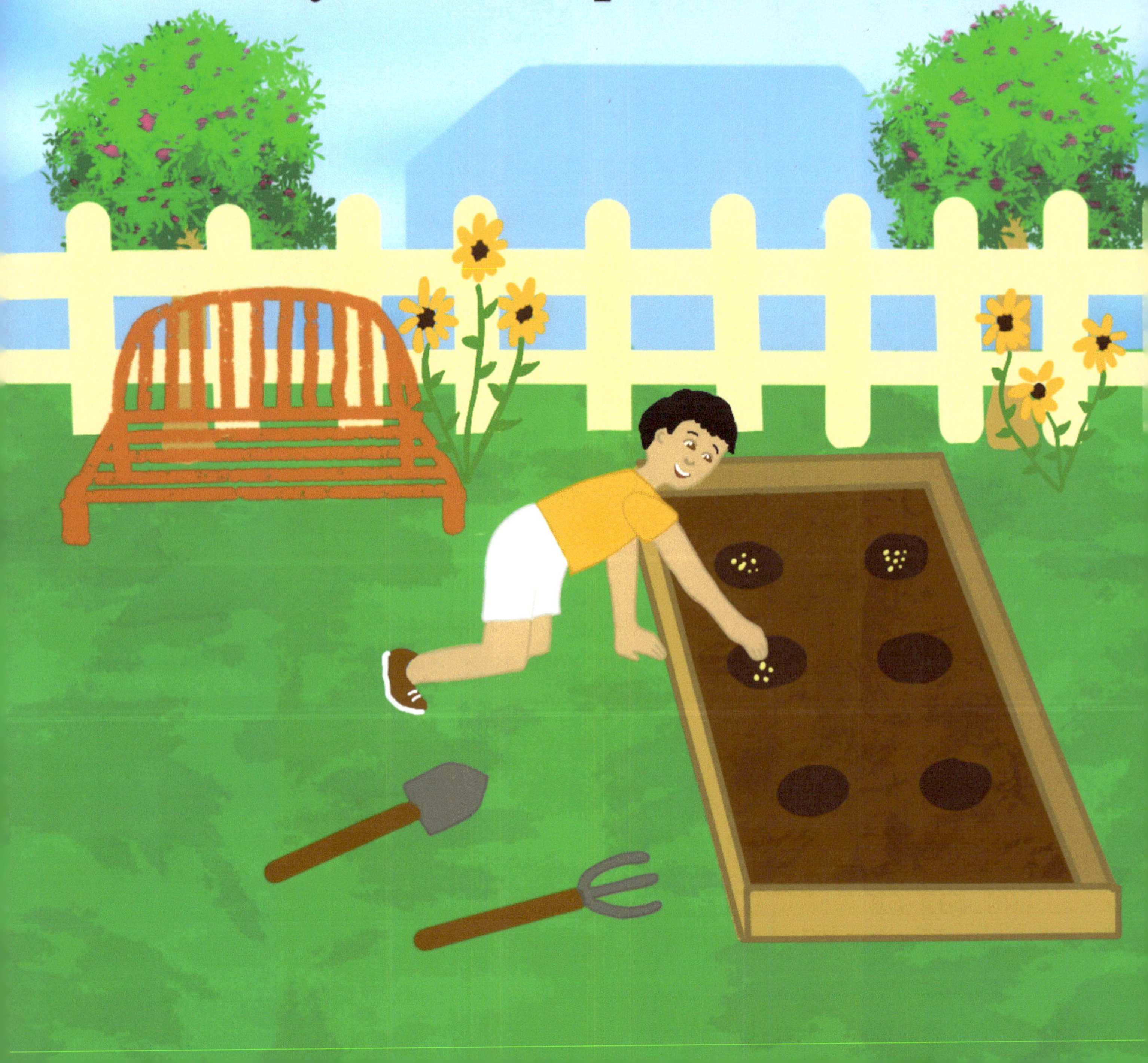

To grow a garden by the trees

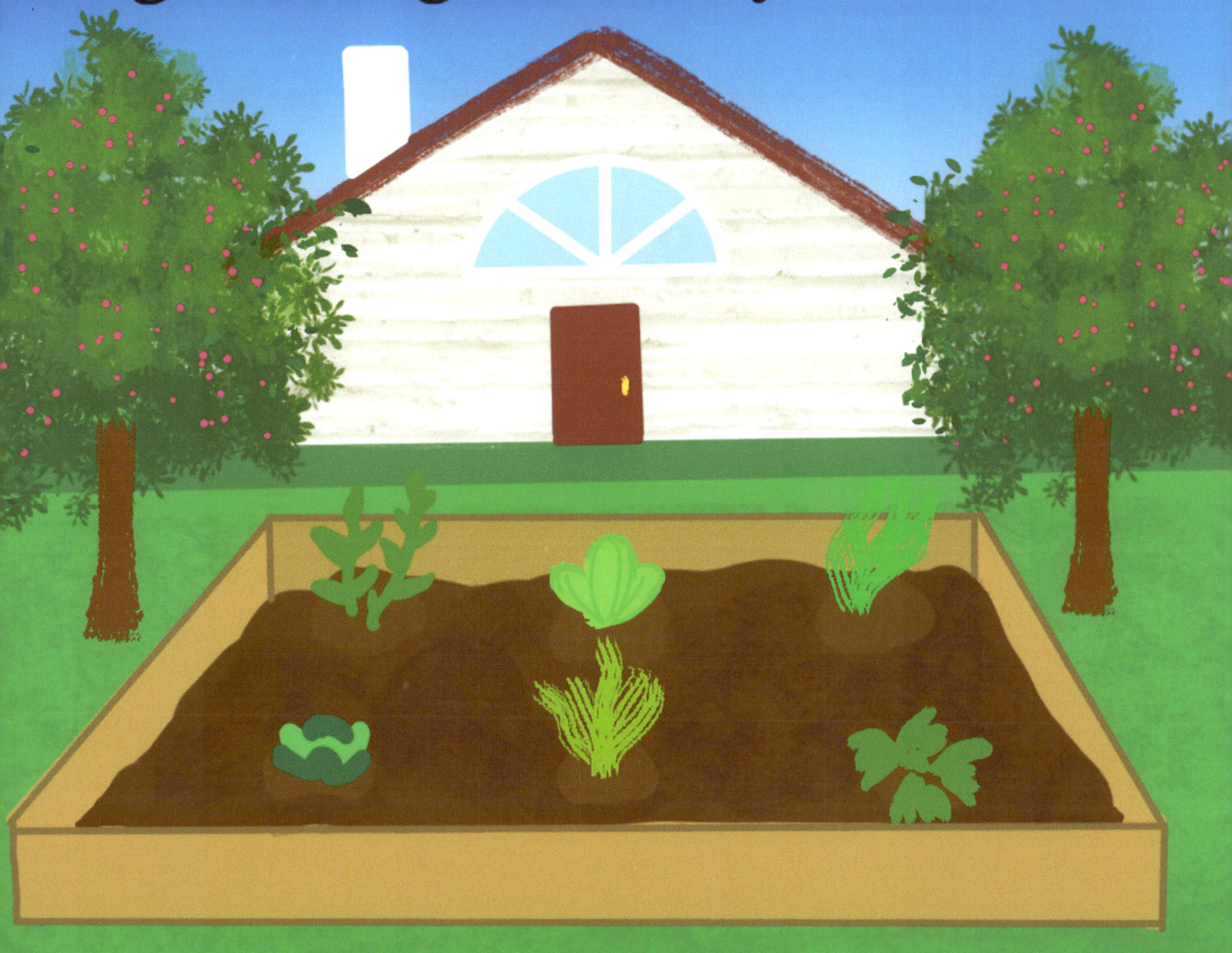

To eat some fruits and veggies too.
It's food that is so good for you.

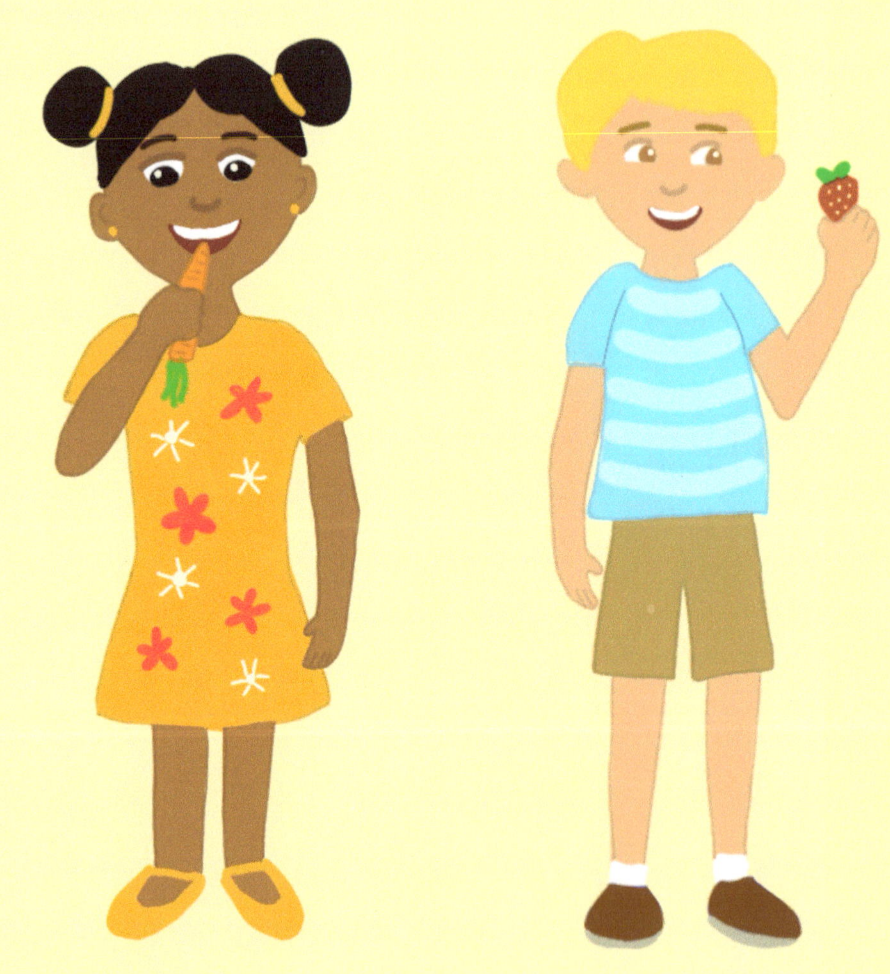

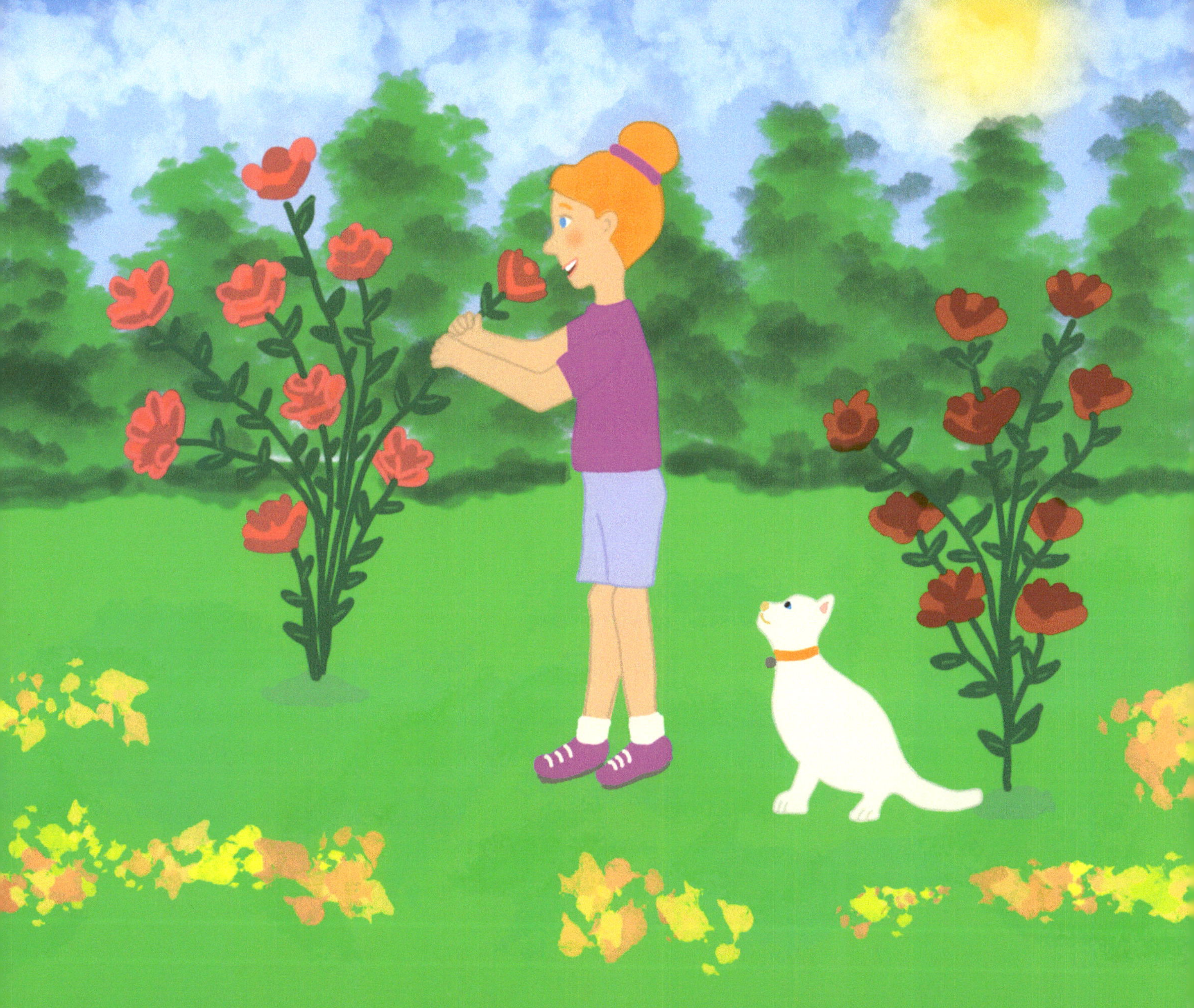

And I'll stop to smell the pretty flowers
Then enjoy Mother Nature for an hour

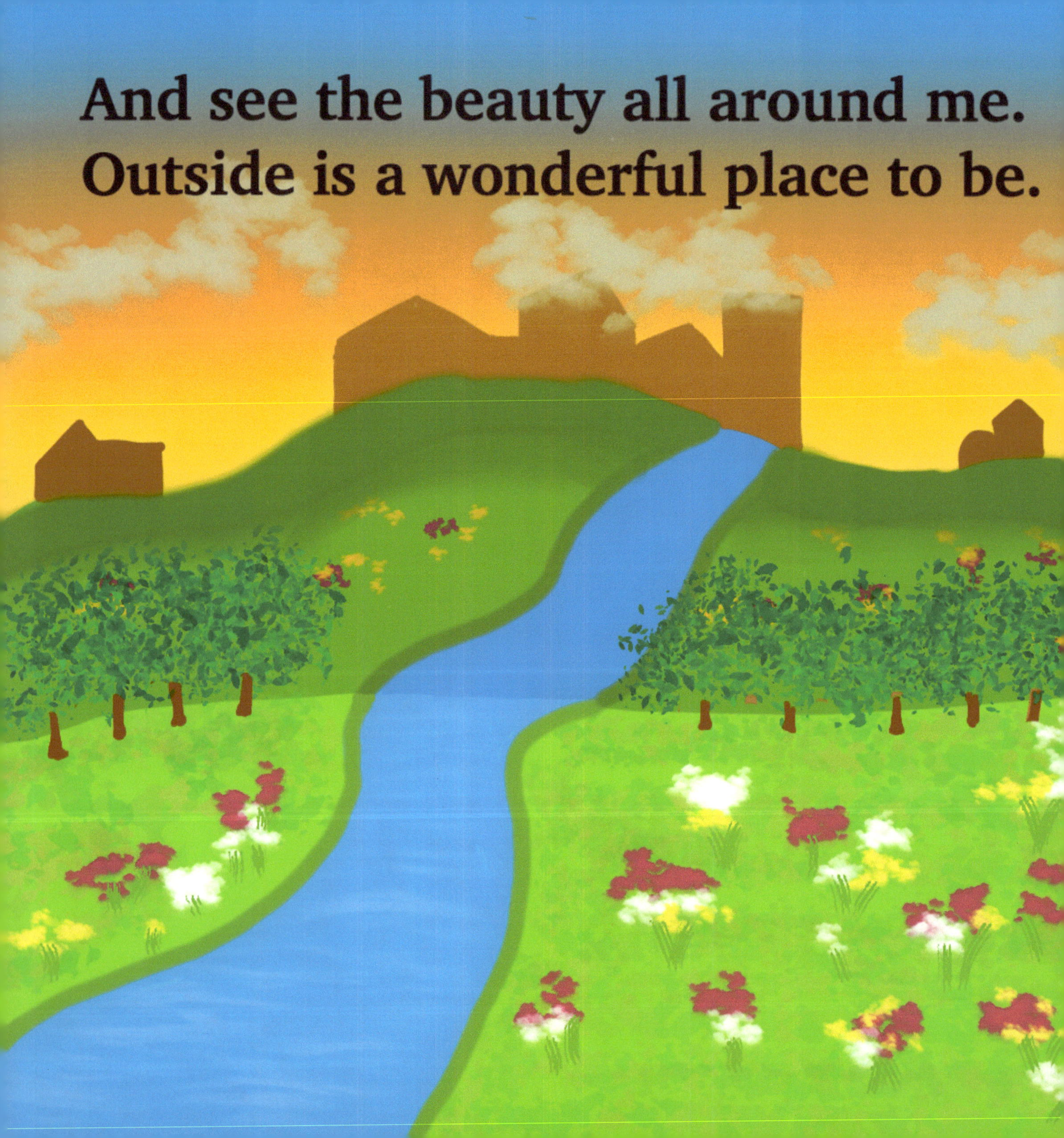

And see the beauty all around me.
Outside is a wonderful place to be.

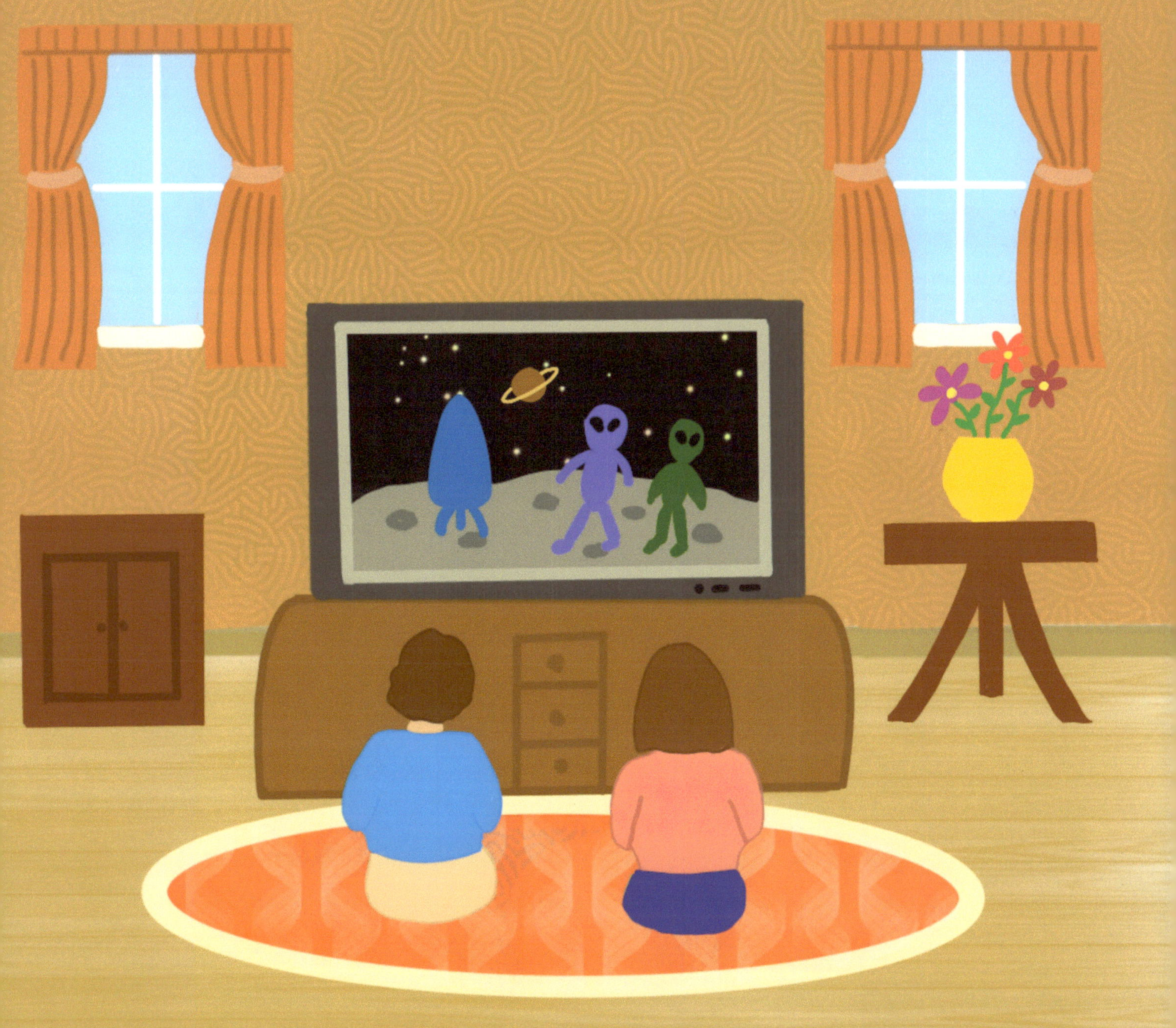

So there is no need to sit around

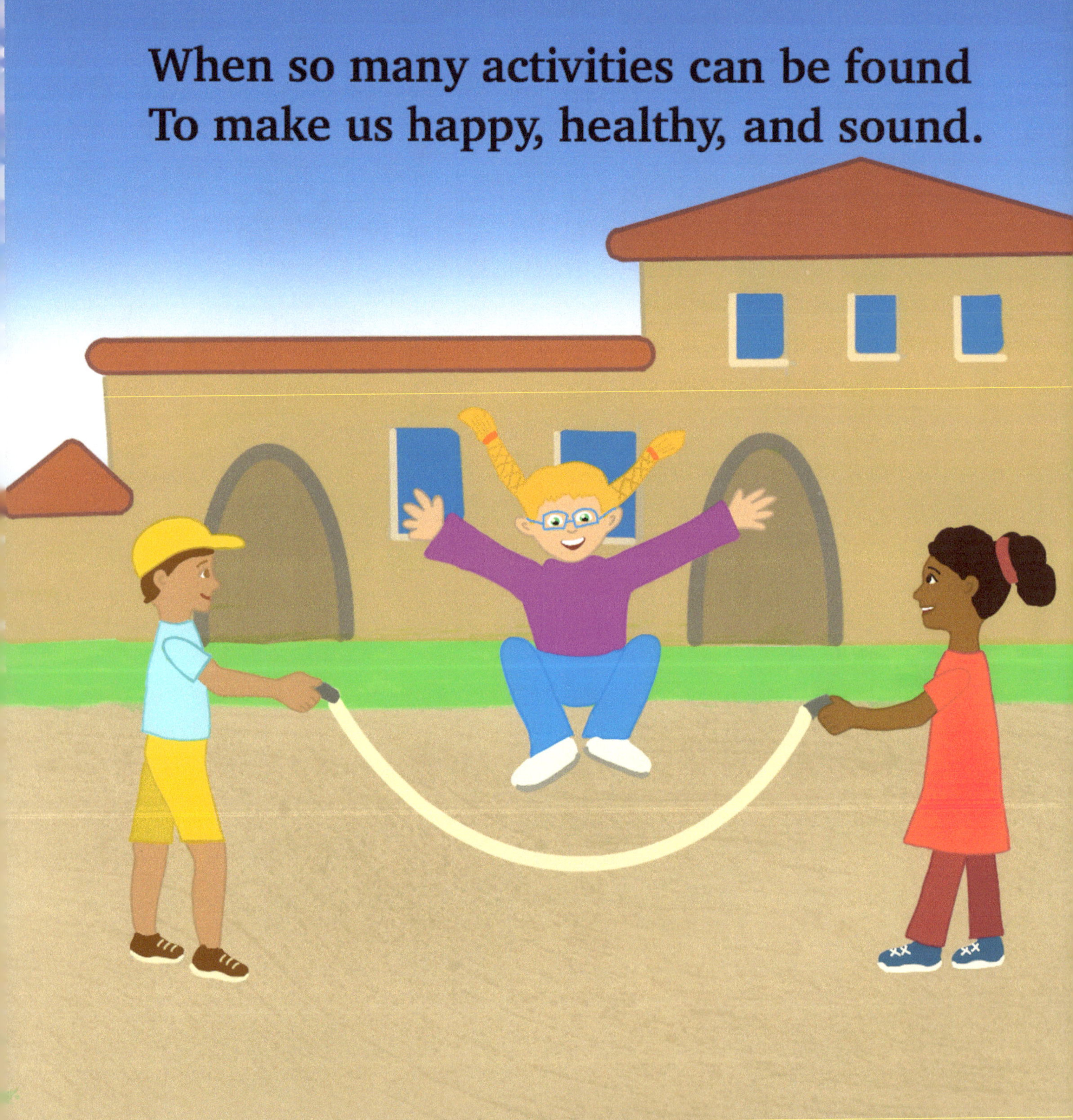

When so many activities can be found
To make us happy, healthy, and sound.

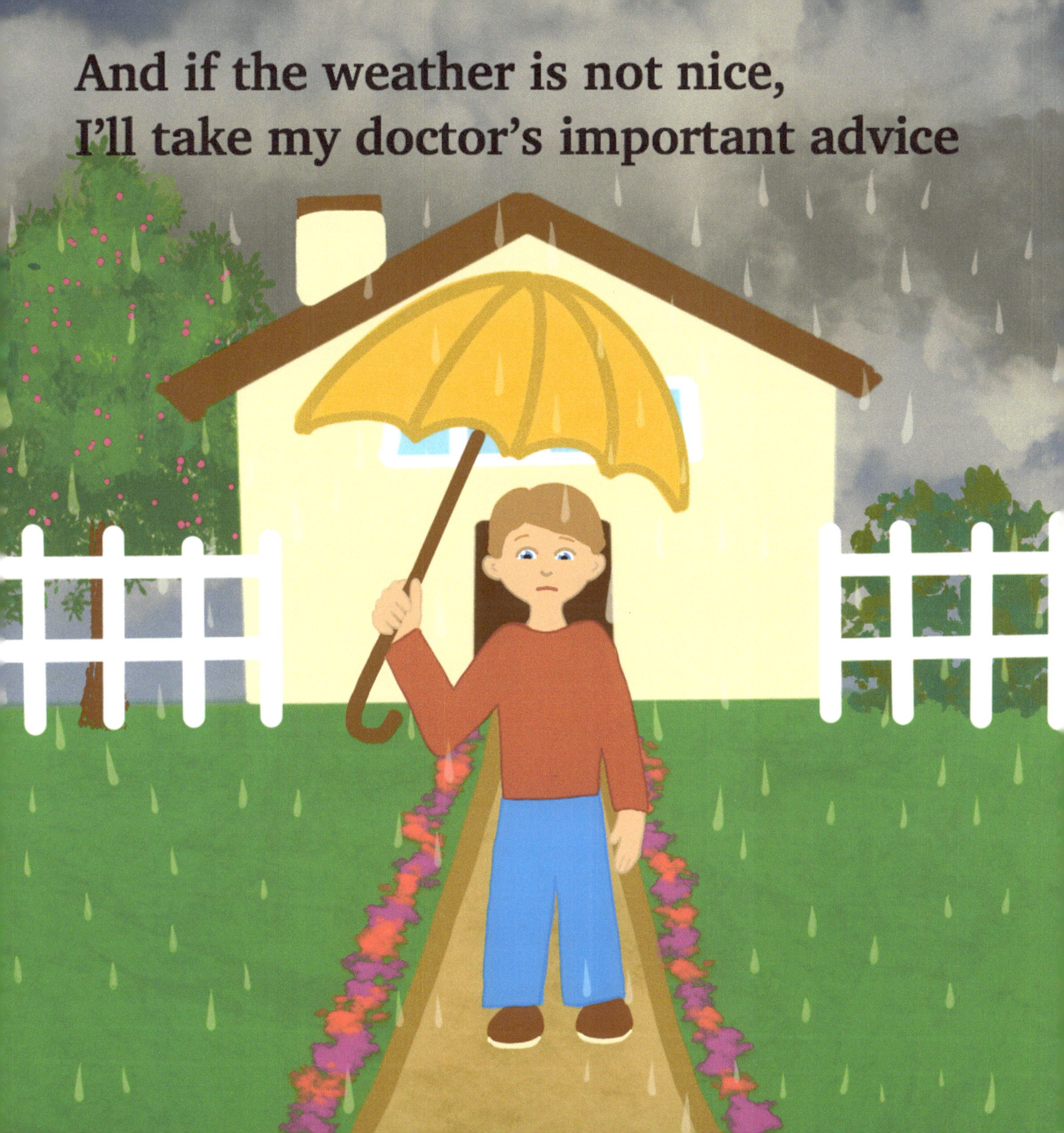

And if the weather is not nice,
I'll take my doctor's important advice

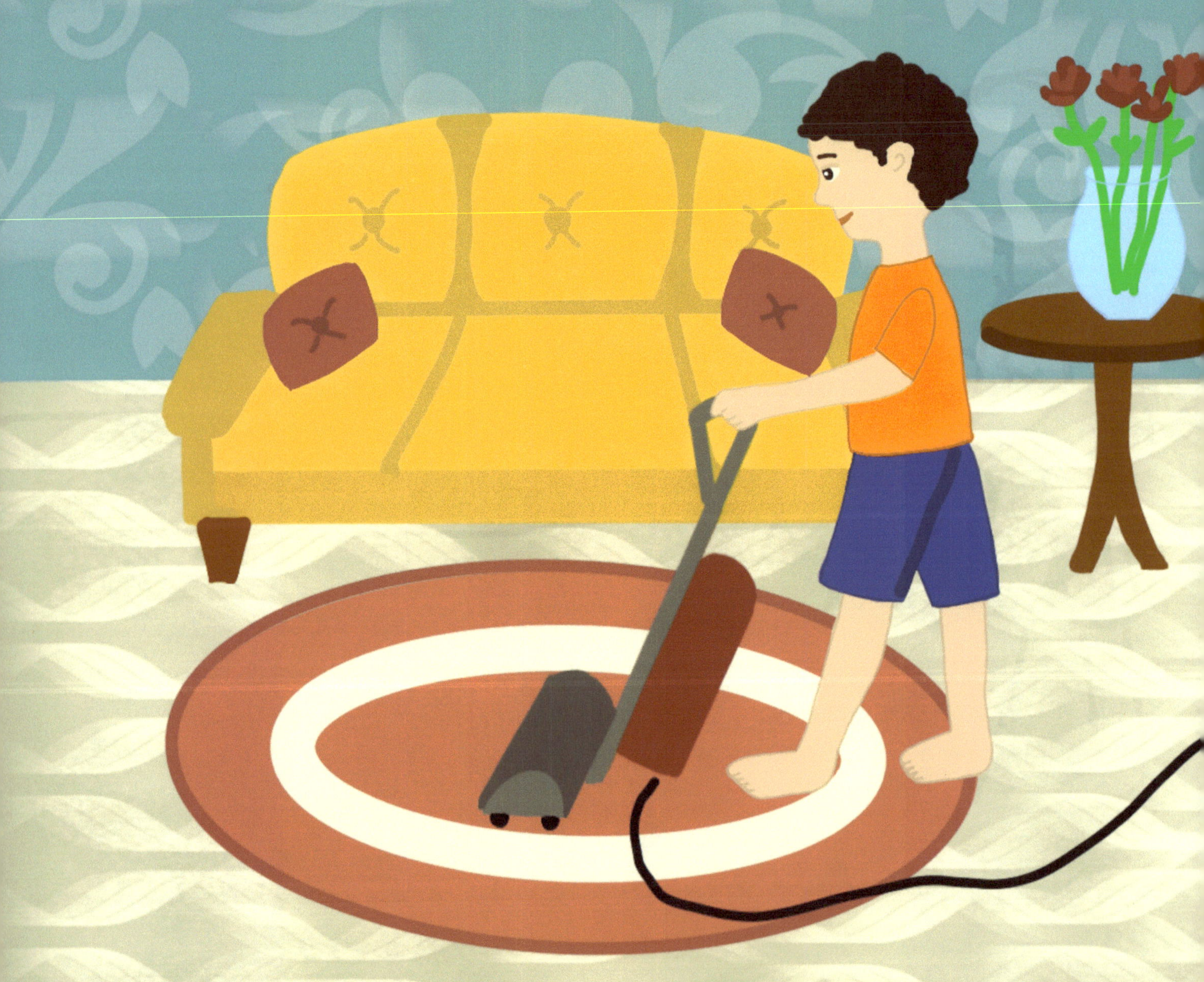

To stay active simply anywhere.
Just get up and move off that chair!

It's such a beautiful day outside!
I hope that now you can decide

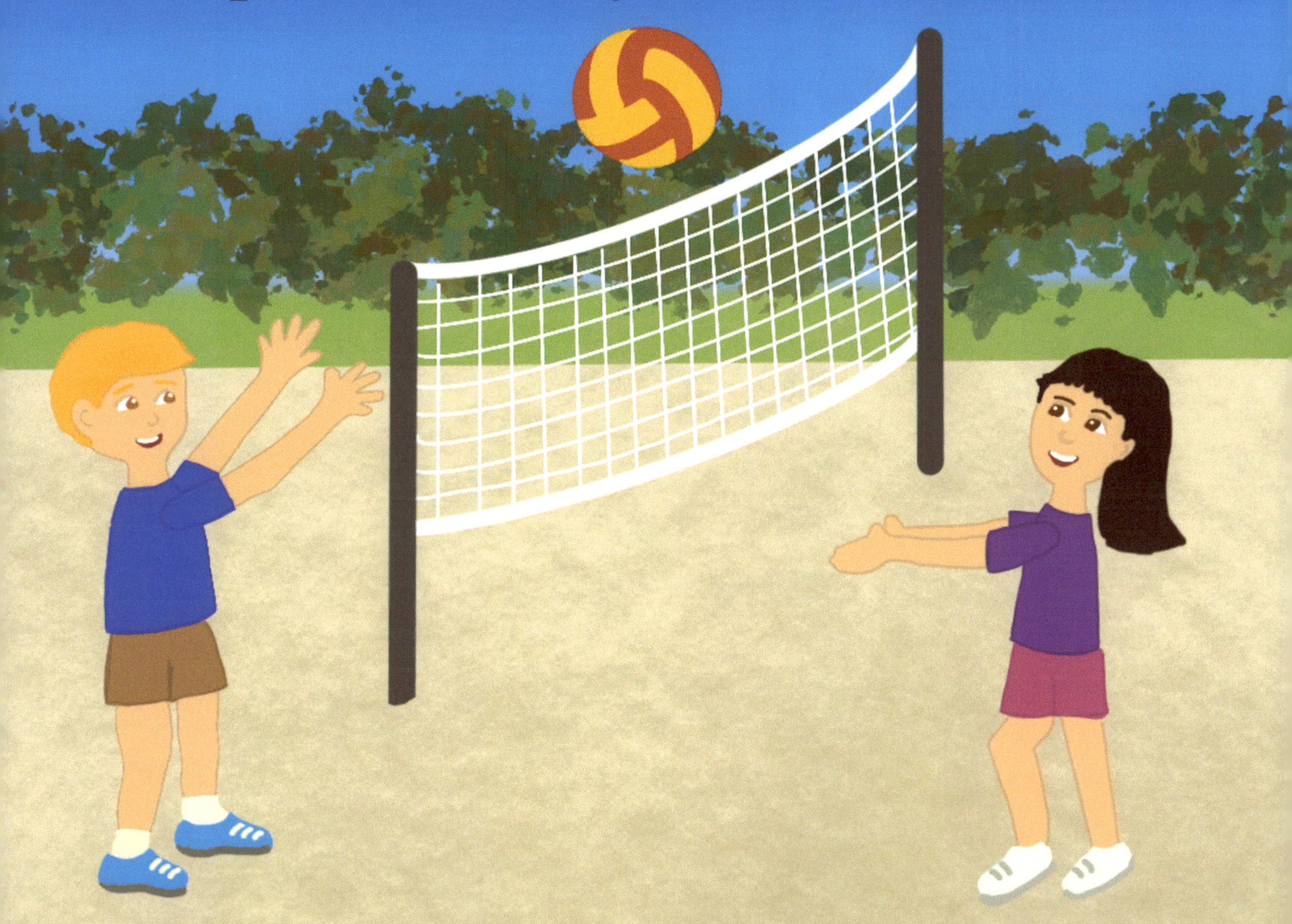

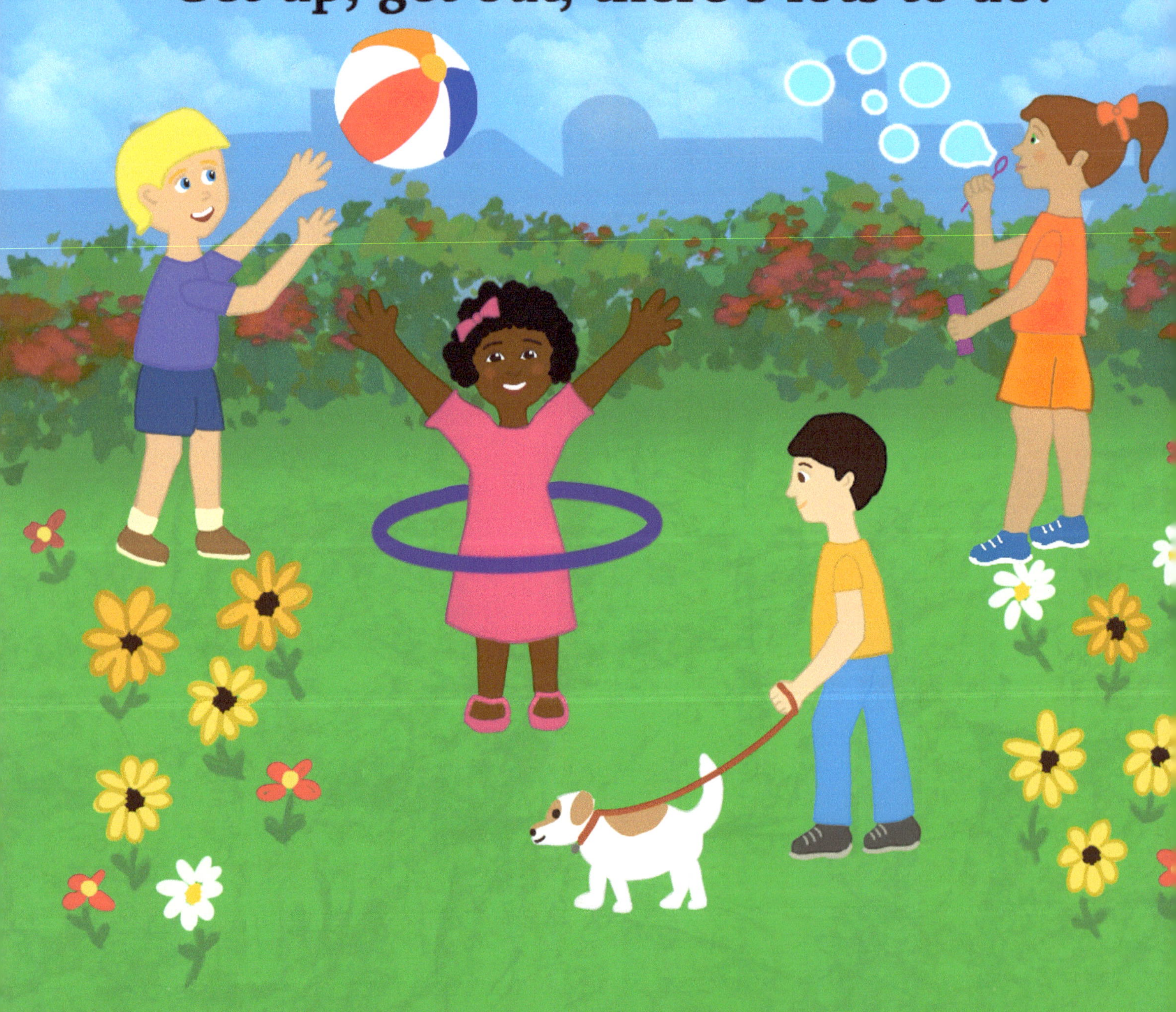

To move around and have fun too.
Get up, get out, there's lots to do!